Basic Concepts of Immunology

An Illustrated Short Course

Basic Concepts of Immunology

An Illustrated Short Course

Deepak K Saini
PhD
Department of Biotechnology
All India Institute of Medical Sciences
New Delhi

Deepti Saini
Department of Biochemistry
All India Institute of Medical Sciences
New Delhi

PEEPEE
PUBLISHERS and DISTRIBUTORS (P) LTD.

Basic Concepts of Immunology—An Illustrated Short Course

Published by
Pawaninder P. Vij

Peepee Publishers and Distributors (P) Ltd.
Head Office: 160, Shakti Vihar, Pitam Pura
Delhi - 110 034 (India)

Correspondence Address:

7/31, First Floor
Ansari Road, Daryaganj, Post Box-7243
New Delhi-110 002 (India)

Ph: 65195868, 23246245, 9811156083

e-mail: peepee160@yahoo.co.in

e-mail: peepee160@rediffmail.com

e-mail: peepee160@gmail.com

www.peepeepub.com

First Edition: 2004
Reprint: **2009**

ISBN: 81-88867-17-9

Printed at
Lordson, C-5/19, Rana Pratap Bagh, Delhi-110007

Preface

Immunology as a science finds its beginning the very first day the human being is conceived. The protection of foetus from infections through maternal immune system is considered 'very' natural and is a phenomenon which doesn't need an exhaustive training in science to understand. Though the science of this immune recognition and reaction is termed as '*Immunology*', the field has broadened its horizons in a very short span and now involves almost every discipline of modern biology and medicine viz. recombinant DNA technology, (genetic engineering), oncology, diagnostics, therapy, genomics, proteomics to name a few. Though it is impossible to discuss all these new areas in the context of this book, some of these disciplines are described with minor details to interest readers towards modern immunology.

We are not expecting that this book will compete with various other excellent immunology textbooks which provide outstanding details and insight in immunology. Rather, we hope that this book will serve as a quick 'insight' cum introductory book for the all students initiating their studies in immunology. Most of the sections in this book are presented with help of diagrams and as points, so that the information is available 'on tips'. To an avid reader the information present in the book might seem too concise and basic, but keeping the objective of this book as a '*Basic Short Course book*', we are hopeful that this book will come in really handy to all readers.

We are grateful to all the people who helped in bringing this book in the current form.

Deepak K Saini
Deepti Saini

Contents

Chapter 1

Immunology—An Overview

Immunology is a complex science which involves study of a battery of cellular and biochemical processes which govern the various phenomena of **recognition** of a non-self entity in the body and **generation of appropriate defense response** to counter that invasion.

Microorganisms present in our surroundings vary to a very large degree and consequently a variety of immune responses are required to counter their attack. Large number of pathogens can be warded off simply by resistance barriers of our body, whereas a few can penetrate these barriers and hence need specialized counter mechanisms. It is the nature of the pathogen and the site of invasion, which essentially determine the type and the strength of the effective immune response. This is on account of differential invasive properties of all the pathogens, no two infections are same and do not manifest same symptoms, hence there have to be a differential counter mechanism for each pathogen from the body as well.

When an effective immune response is mounted the individual remains disease free and disease occurs in case of failure of an effective immune response. However, under certain situations and conditions, the immune response can lead to deviations as mentioned below.

1. **Autoimmunity** – Term given to mistaken recognition of self-proteins or entities as foreign. This leads to generation of an

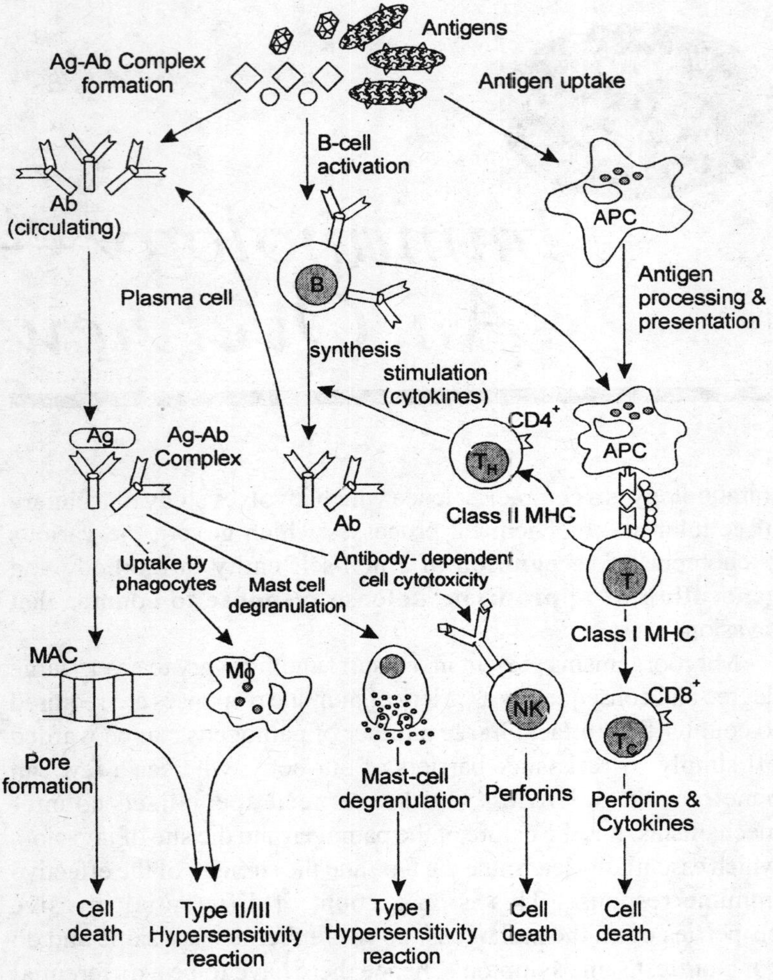

Figure 1.1. Type of immune responses.

immune response against 'self' tissues and cells and generate a reaction against them. Such disorders include disease like rheumatoid arthritis and pernicious anemia. These disorders are discussed in detail in Chapter 8.

2. **Immunodeficiency** – A more severe form of immunological deviation wherein the body fails to elicit an effective immune response against foreign antigens, due to some defect in the immune system. In such cases, the individual is hypersusceptible to any kind of infection. Such disorders are either inborn, e.g. SCID (severe combined immunodeficiency disorder) or generated afterwards as a result of infection from HIV which leads to development of AIDS (acquired immunodeficiency syndrome). Such conditions are also discussed in Chapter 8.

3. **Hypersensitivity** – The third deviation of the immune response is also the most common deviation and is seen in almost every individual in one form or another. Termed as hypersensitivity it is essentially an outcome of an overactive immune response. This happens when immune cells recognize a less toxic or less reactive foreign molecule *viz.* a food molecule, dust, pollen grains, etc. as a very harmful pathogen and hence elicit an exaggerated response which consequently causes more damage than the pathogen or the molecule. Such responses include disorders like asthma, wheal and flare reaction, hay fever to name a few.

Chapter 2

Innate and Acquired Immunity

The 'immune response' which counters the invasion gets into action at many distinct sites and through various modes. These sites (or organs) are classified on the basis of their role in generation of immune response.

1. The primary site which initially encounters the invasion from the microorganisms is the epithelia, which forms the first line of barrier for *innate immunity*, e.g. skin, mucosal lining of the nasal pathway, eye, GI tract, urogenital tract, etc. These systems protect the body by their 'barrier' like action, which is present right from birth and hence are nonadaptive response.
   - These barriers cannot recognize or discriminate different foreign entities and hence cannot mount a specific immune response. Since invasion from the tough lysosome-rich skin is rather difficult, the majority of the infections come through penetration, colonization and adhesion of the microorganism to the internal mucosal lining of the body.
   - Besides these physical barriers a number of immune cells also form part of the innate immunity mechanism like phagocytic macrophages, which bind the bacterium through their surface adhesions and engulf them, leading to production of biologically active immune effector molecules called as '*cytokines*', which can affect the immunogical outcome of the surrounding cells which bear the receptors for them.

They also produce other chemoattractant molecules called as *'chemokines'* which attract the cells like neutrophils and basophils from the blood to the site of infection to initiate the process of inflammation.

- The innate immune response also makes a very critical and crucial contribution to the adaptive immunity process. The inflammatory response increases the net turnover of the blood flow at the site of infection hence increasing the recruitment of antigen presenting cells and lymphoid cells.

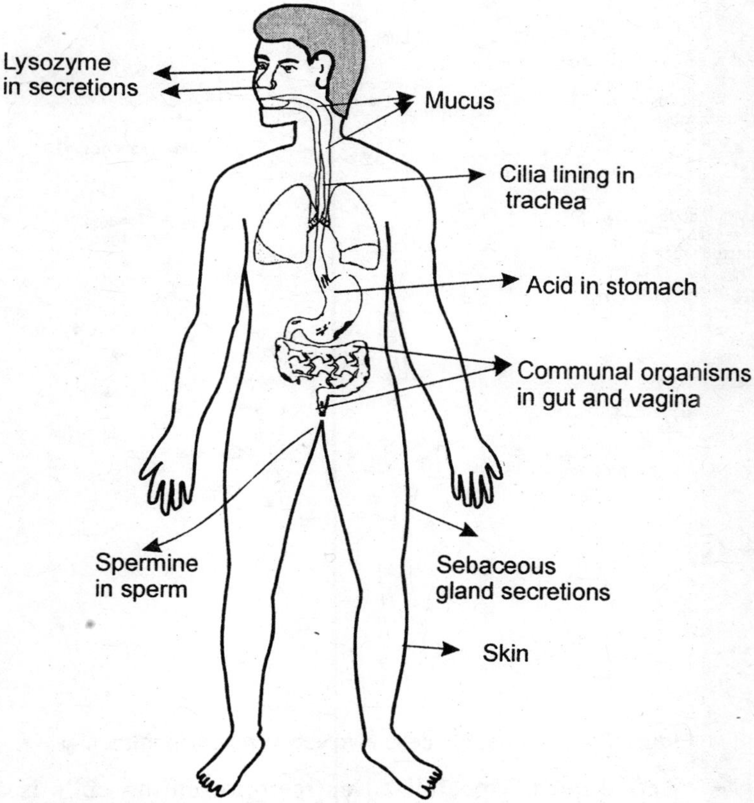

Figure 2.1: Exterior defences working through innate immunity

2. The secondary sites which generate an **adaptive immunity** response harbor specialized cells which counter an invasion process. Such organs include lymph nodes, thymus, spleen, tonsils, bone marrow, etc.

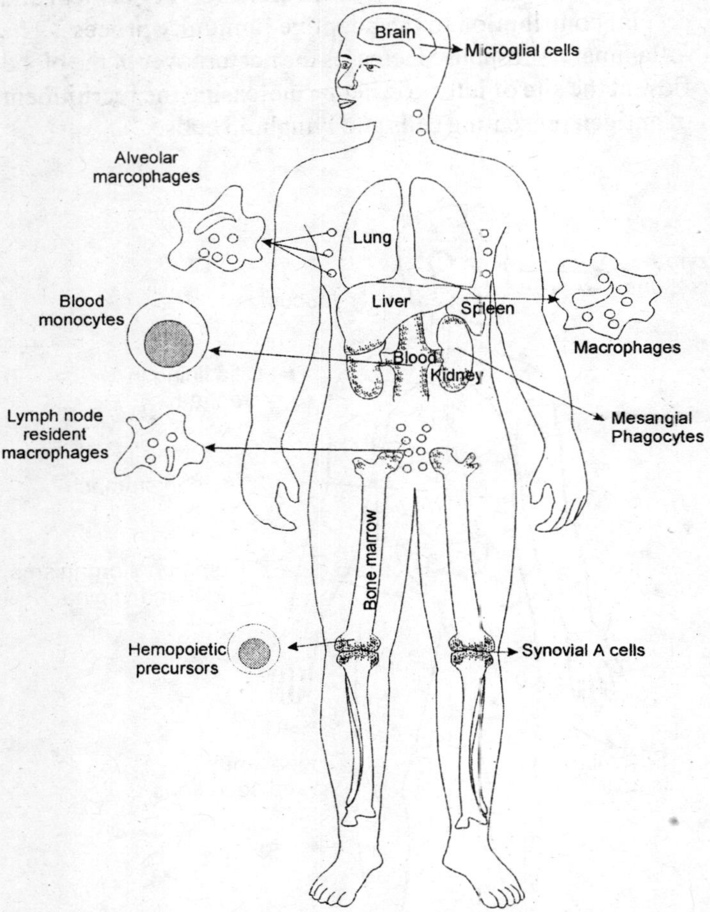

Figure 2.2: Organs and cells involved in adaptive immunity

- Activation of specialized antigen-presenting cells is a necessary first step for induction of adaptive immunity. This process is performed by specialized cells such as dendritic cells and macrophages amongst others.

- The activated antigen-presenting cells ingest the antigen, process it and present it to the lymphocytes to activate them, which give rise to clones of antigen-specific cells that mediate adaptive immunity. Hence, the 'clonal selection process' is central to the process of adaptive immunity.

The essential differences in innate and adaptive responses are listed below.

Feature	Adaptive immunity	Innate immunity
Development (after)	Initial exposure	Birth
Mediators	Cells	Anatomic barriers and non-specific immune cells
Specificity	Highly specific	Non-specific memory
of pathogen	Present	Not present
Enhancement	Possible through vaccination	Not possible

I. ORGANS OF IMMUNE RESPONSE

A number of organs are involved in generation of an effective immune response and they are essentially divided in (i) central and (ii) peripheral lymphoid organs.

1. **Central lymphoid organs**—Organs wherein immuno-competent cells develop viz.
   a. Bone marrow – Site of origin of immune cells and B-cell development
   b. Thymus – Site of T-cell development
2. **Peripheral lymphoid organs**—Organs wherein immuno-competency of cells are developed.
   a. Spleen
   b. Lymph nodes
   c. Tonsils
   d. Intestinal Payer's patches
   e. Mucosa

II. CELLS OF THE IMMUNE SYSTEM

A number of cells participate in a direct or indirect manner in generation of a proper immunological reaction in response to an invasion process. These cells are of three basic types – Antigen-presenting cells (**APCs**); thymus derived cells (**T-cells**) and bone marrow-derived cells (**B-cells**) and these cells work in sync to generate two types of immune response:

1. **Humoral immunity** - Mediated through proteins called as antibodies, the pathogen or foreign invader neutralizing entities. The neutralized pathogen is then removed through many cellular processes including phagocytosis or lysis. The antibodies are generated by B – cells through mediation of APCs and T-cells (T_H).
2. **Cell-mediated immunity** –Involves eradication of invading cellular pathogen or malfunctioning self cells through cell lysis. Such a response is mediated by either natural killer (NK) cells, macrophages (Mϕ) or cytotoxic T-cells (T_C).

These two immune recognition and processing phenomena are highly interrelated as evident from the involvement of same cells in two different types of response. It is the interplay of these two immune responses which govern the final outcome of an immune response.

Origin and Development of Immune Cells

- Primarily all immune cells develop from common pleuripotent stem cell present in the bone marrow called as *hematopoietic stem cell*, which differentiates whose into variable types of immune cell progenitors leads to the formation of various effector immune cells in various secondary lymphoid organs.
- The various development stages of these cells can be analyzed using various surface markers expressed on these cells in a highly stage specific manner. Such surface markers which can distinguish these immune cells are called as '*clusters of differentiation*' (CD) markers. For example, T-cells contain CD3 marker whereas B-cells CD19.
- Hematopoietic stem cell differentiates into two major types of WBC progenitors apart from the platelet progenitor cells the *megakaryocyte* and RBC precursor cell, the *erythroblast*.

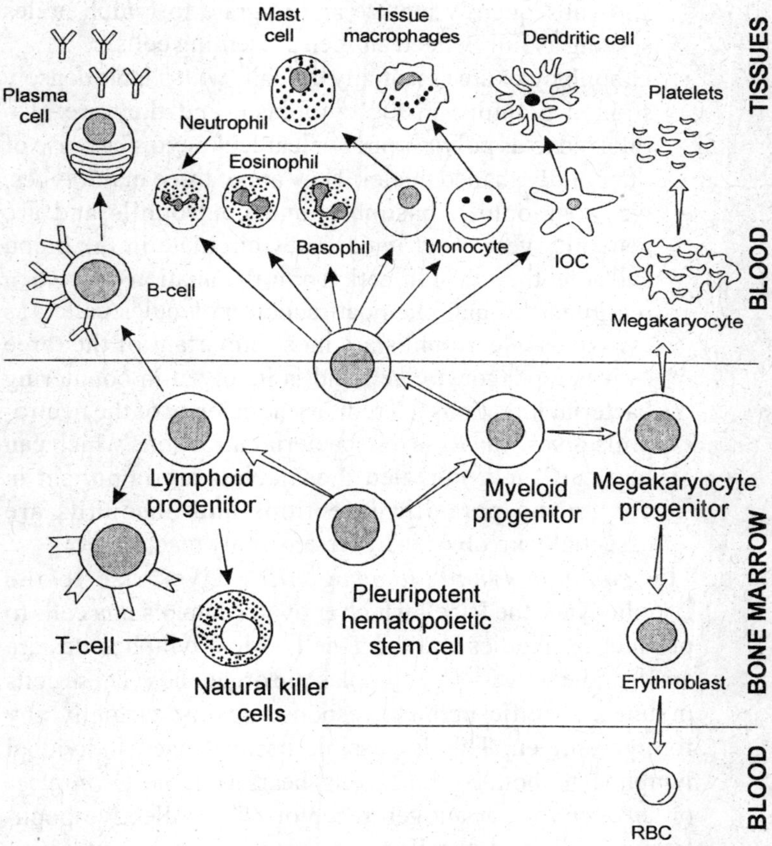

Figure 2.3: Cells of immune system, their origin and development.

a. *Myeloid progenitor* is the precursor of the granulocytes, macrophages, dendritic cells and the mast cells of the immune system.

- Macrophages are one of the important phagocytic cells of the body and are widely distributed as well. They originate from the monocytes, which circulate in the blood and differentiate into macrophages only upon their migration into tissues.
- Dendritic cells are specialized antigen-processing cells. They reside in the tissues where they ingest the antigen

and subsequently mature and migrate to lymph nodes serving as full fledged antigen presenting cells.

- Granulocytes are essentially the cells which have densely stained granules in the cytoplasm and they are also referred to as polymorphonuclear leukocytes because of their oddly shaped nuclei. They are of three major types, *viz.* eosinophils, basophils and neutrophils and are generally very short lived. They circulate in the blood and enter the site of infection or inflammation only when recruited through chemoattractant molecules called as cytokines. Neutrophils are most important of the three as it is a phagocytic cell and is involved in countering bacterial infections. Hereditary deficiency of the neutrophils gives way to severe bacterial infections which can be fatal if left untreated. Eosinophils are important in countering parasitic infections and basophils are essentially involved in hypersensitivity reactions.

b. The *common lymphoid progenitor* gives rise to the lymphocytes, the B-cell which activates into plasma cells to produce antibodies and the T-cells. Most lymphocytes are small and with very few cytoplasmic organelles. These cells mount a specific immune response against virtually any foreign antigen. This is possible because each individual lymphocyte (both B- and T-cells) bears a unique *'prototype'* or *'progenitor'* of antigen receptor. The collective populations of B- and T-cells hence have a huge repertoire of receptors that are highly diverse in antigen-binding sites.

- A third type of lymphoid cells originating from the common lymphoid progenitor is called as the natural killer cell. Unlike the other lymphoid cells, these cells do not have the antigen recognition receptors on their surface and are a better suited component of the innate immune system. They are able to recognize and kill abnormal cells like tumor cells and virally-infected cells.

Development of Lymphocytes

- The development of the lymphocytes takes place in the lymphoid organs wherein the lymphocytes mature in a mesh of non-lymphocytic cells.

- The interaction between the lymphocytic and non-lymphocytic cells is very essential for development, initiation and sustenance of immune response.
- It is here in the lymphoid organs the lymphocytes learn to discriminate between self and foreign antigens. Any antigen encountered during the course of development of antigen-discrimination process of lymphocytes is treated as self and non-further immune response to the same is generated.
- The B- and T-lymphocytes which have matured in the bone marrow and thymus but have not encountered any antigen yet are termed as naïve lymphocytes. These cells continuously circulate in the blood from where they enter the peripheral lymphoid tissues and return to the blood via the lymphatic vessels. In case of an encounter with the antigen (through infection) they are 'arrested' in the lymphoid tissues, where they proliferate and differentiate into effector cells capable of combating and neutralizing the infection.

  a. *Development of B-cells:* B-cells essentially develop in the bone marrow and achieve maturity in the peripheral lymphoid organs. The stages in the B-cells development are distinguished by the expression of immunoglobulin chains and specific cell-surface proteins (CD). The first classification of the B-cell lineage in different development stages was made according to their immunoglobulin chain expression status i.e. whether no chain is expressed or only heavy chain is expressed or both the chains are expressed. Later, intermediate differentiation stages have been distinguished on the basis of the expression of other cell surface proteins. All development upto the immature B-cell takes place in the bone marrow and is essentially antigen independent (Table 2.1).

  b. *Development of T-cells:* T-cells develop from a common lymphoid progenitor in the bone marrow and the subsequent differentiation into naïve or effector T-cells takes place in the thymus.

Table 2.1: Features of B – cell lineage

Development stage	*H-chain genes*	*L-chain genes*	*Surface Ig*	*CD markers*
Stem cell	Germline	Germline	Absent	CD34, CD45
Early pro- B-cell	D-J rearrangement	Germline	Absent	CD34, CD19, CD45, CD43, CD10, CD38
Late pro B – cell	V-DJ rearrangement	Germline	Absent	CD10, CD19, CD45R, CD43, CD24,CD25, CD40
Large pre- B-cell	VDJ rearranged	Germline	Intracellular m chain	CD19, CD20, CD45R, CD43, CD24, CD-25, CD38
Small pre- B-cell	VDJ rearranged	VJ rearranging	Intracellular m chain	CD19, CD20, CD38, CD45, CD24
Immature B-cell	VDJ rearranged	VJ rearranged	IgM expressed on cell surface	CD19, CD20, CD40, CD45
Mature naïve B-cell	VDJ rearranged	VJ rearranged	IgM and IgD expressed	CD19, CD20, CD40. CD45R
Lymphoblast	VDJ rearranged	VJ rearranged secreted μ chains	IgM secreted	CD19, CD20, CD21, CD40, CD45R
Memory B-cell	Isotype switching to γ, α or ε chains and somatic mutations	VJ rearranged, somatic hypermutations	IgD on cell surface	CD19, CD20, CD21, CD40, CD45R
Plasma cell	Isotype switching to γ, α or ε chains	VJ rearranged	Secreted Ig	CD38 and plasma cell antigen -1

- *Most developing T-cells die in the thymus*: The T-cell precursors arriving in the thymus from the bone-marrow spend upto a week differentiating before they enter a phase of intense proliferation. One an average only about 2 – 5 % of T-cells mature to leave thymus. The rest of the cells die in the thymus by apoptosis and the dying cells are rapidly cleared off by the resident macrophages in the thymic cortex to maintain the smooth flow of the T-cell traffic in thymus. This prolific waste of T-cells in the thymus is an integral process which involves screening of each T-cell for its ability to recognize self-MHC and its ability to discriminate between self- and non-self antigen by inducing self-tolerance.
- *T-cell development stages are marked change in the cell-surface markers* (CD markers): Developing thymocytes undergo a series of distinct phases which are marked by the changes in the status of the T-cell receptor genes and in the expression of TCR along with the changes in the expression of 'many' cell surface marker proteins such as the CD4 complex and the selection of co-receptor proteins CD4 and CD8. These surface changes mark the functional maturation of the T-cell. Hence, particular combinations of cell surface proteins (the CD antigens) thus can be used as markers for T-cells at different stages of differentiation.
- In general, the T-cell development stages are marked on the basis of their major discriminating surface markers the CD4 and CD8 antigen. Since, the CD4 and CD8 makers discriminate the final effector T_H and T_C cells, the development stages of the T-cells are marked on the basis of the presence of these markers. The major stages are:

a. *ble negative cells:* At this stage the T-cell does not ress CD4 or CD8 marker ($CD4^-$ and $CD8^-$) hence *ouble – negative*'. They are generated immediately after try of differentiation of T-cell progenitor in thymus. These mature double negative T-cells can differentiate into either αβ T-cells which form the $CD4^+$ or $CD8^+$ T-cells or they can also form a small population of γδ T-cells.

b. *Double positive cells:* The double negative T-cells undergo gene rearrangement, maturation and differentiation in the thymus only to form pre-T-cell receptor (TCR) and express both CD4 and CD8 markers, hence '*double positive*'. These double positive cells undergo MHC-recognition training in thymus. The cells which can recognize the self-MHC undergo 'positive selection' and undergo maturation to express higher levels of TCR. Other (majority) cells which cannot recognize the self-MHC and recognize the self-antigens undergo 'negative selection' and die. Only upto 2 % of the double positive cells survive this screening process and mature further.

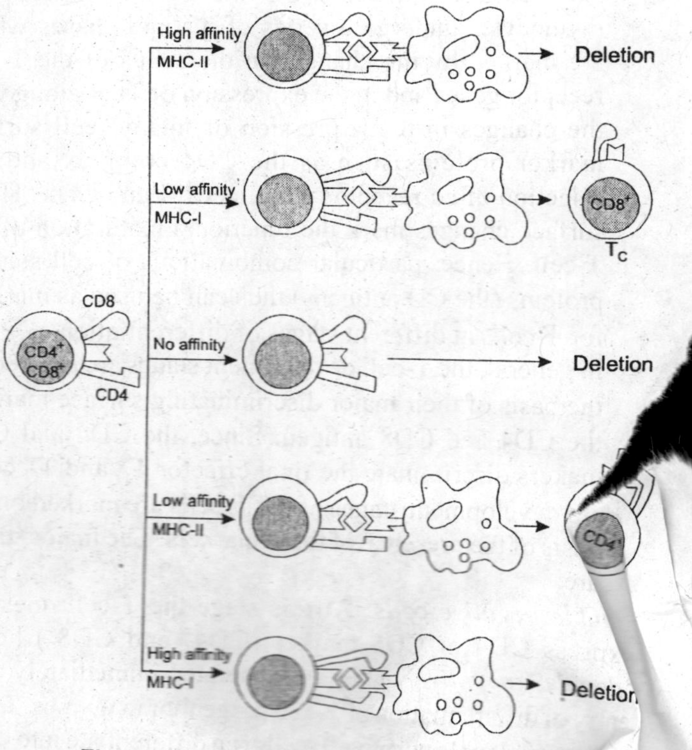

Figure 2.4: Recognition of self-MHC by T-cells

c. *Single positive cells* – After the successful positive and negative selection process the cells which survive express only one of the receptor molecules from CD4 or CD8 receptors, becoming either $CD4^+$ or $CD8^+$ *single-positive* thymocytes (Fig. 2.4).

Table 2.2: Features of T-cell lineage

Site / Location	*T-cell development stage*	*β-chain/α-chain status of TCR*	*Surface markers*
Bone marrow	Stem Cell	Germline/ germline	CD34?
Thymus	Early double negative thymocyte	DJ rearranged/ germline	CD2, CD44
	Late double negative thymocyte	VDJ rearranged/ germline	CD25, CD44, HSA
	Early double positive thymocyte	VDJ rearranged/ VJ rearranged	CD4, CD8, Pre– Tα
	Late double – positive thymocyte	VDJ rearranged/ VJ rearranged	CD4, CD8, CD69
Peripheral lymphoid organs	Naïve $CD4^+$ T-cell		CD4, CD62, CD45RA, CD5
	Memory $CD4^+$ T-cell		CD4, CD45RO, CD44
	Effector $CD4^+$ T-cell		CD4, CD45RO, CD44
	Naïve $CD8^+$ T-cell		CD8, CD45RA
	Memory $CD8^+$ T-cell		CD8, CD45RO, CD44
	Effector $CD8^+$ T-cell		CD8, CD44

III. THE COMPLEMENT SYSTEM

- Complement consists of a group of serum proteins that activate each other in an orderly fashion to generate biologically active molecules, enzymes, opsonins, anaphylotoxins and chemotoxins. They are called as 'complement' because of their ability to complement the antibacterial activities of antibodies.

- The complement fixation results in cell lysis and requires 9 major factors – C1 to C9, majority of which are zymogens, which are essentially proteases which are activated by proteolytic cleavage.
- Since complement pathways are not entirely dependent on the cellular immune response or the cells of the immune system, it forms an essential component of the innate immune response.
- Complement can be activated via three processes.
  1. The **classical pathway** which is initiated by Ag-Ab complex which activates the C1q protein of the C1 complex. Once the C1 complex is activated it leads to activation of C4 followed by C2 and C3 proteins and consequently the initial C3 convertase complex is generated.
  2. The **alternative pathway** in which the complement components become activated by the cell wall of some bacteria and yeasts in combination with serum factors B and D and properdin. Since it was discovered as an 'alternative' pathway of complement activation from the classical pathway it is called as alternative pathway. Technically it is pathogen activated complement fixation pathway.
  3. The **mannan-binding lecithin pathway** is very similar to the classical pathway as it uses a protein highly similar to C1q protein the MBL which is a collectin. The MBL complex binds to the pathogen surface to activate two zymogens MASP-1 and MASP-2 which lead to proteolytic activation of C4 and C2 protein and consequential activation of the complement fixation pathway.
- The complement activation is largely confined to the surface on which it is activated as most of the activation reactions involve covalent bonding of one of the activated components to the complex. This helps in preventing the diffusion of proteins to other sites and hence increases the local concentration of the components to facilitate focused and localized attack (Fig. 2.5).
- The level of complement does not increase after immunization and its activity and components is tightly regulated by various inhibitors.

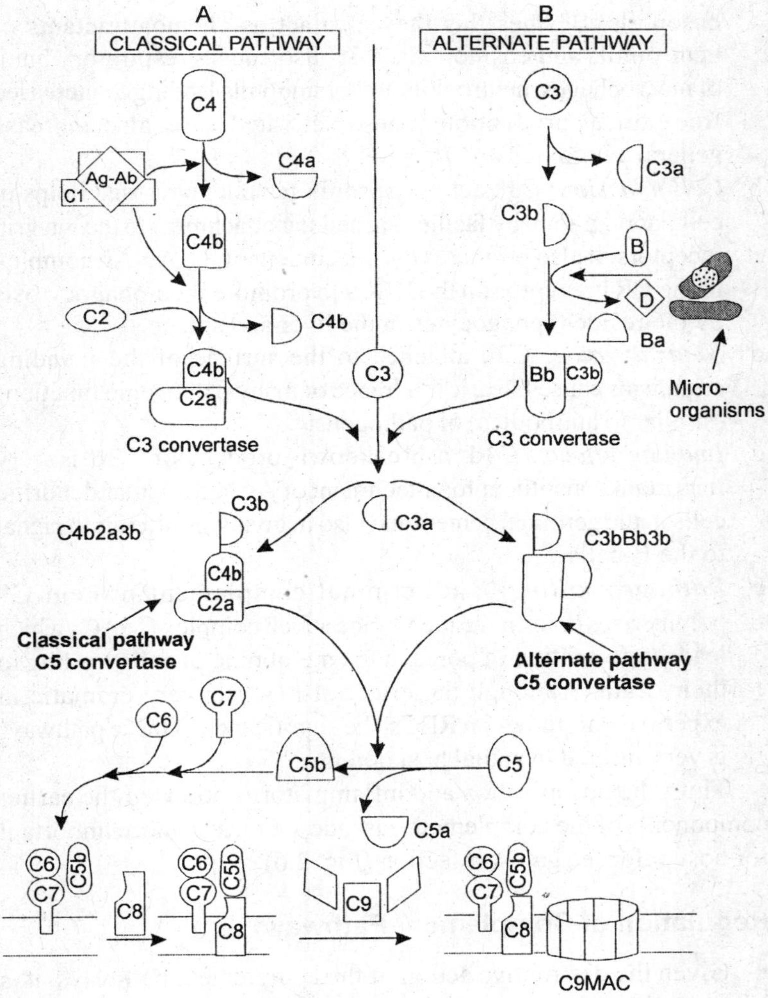

Figure 2.5: Complement activation pathways

Functions of Complement

a. *Pro inflammatory effects:* C3a and C5a complement proteins act as anaphylotoxins and cause degranulation of mast cells and basophils. Besides this they also act as chemoattractants of neutrophils and eosinophils. C3b also causes respiratory burst of macrophages, neutrophils and eosinophils leading to increased free radical production. These activated cells also increase general cytotoxicity.

b. *Cell adhesion:* C3b acts as opsonin for phagocytosis; helps in cellular migration by facilitating cellular attachment to the integrin receptors. It also promotes the attachment of the Ag-Ab complex to the CR1 receptor on the RBCs to promote their phagocytosis by the resident phagocytes in the liver and spleen.
c. *Neutralization:* C3b attached to the surface of the invading organisms causes stearic hindrance of many pathogenic functions (similar to antibodies) of pathogens.
d. *Immune effects*: C3d, a breakdown product of C3b is very important constituent for attachment of Ag to follicular dendritic cells in the germinal centers and also in giving proliferation signal to the B-cells.
e. *Pathogen killing*: The terminal complement protein C9 polymerizes to form the membrane attack complex (MAC) which leads to formation of pores in the membrane of cells leading to their death. Although the effect of MAC is very dramatic in experimental studies on RBCs, the significance of these pathways is very limited in actual host defense.

Thus, the opsonization and inflammatory actions of the earlier components of the complement cascade are clearly more important for host defense against infection (Fig. 2.6).

Regulation of Complement Pathways

- Given the destructive action of the complement pathways, it is very critical to have the entire pathway tightly regulated to prevent its uncontrolled activation.
- The activation of complement proteins is regulated by a series of host proteins such as
  a. *Serpin*, which regulates the C1 activation (also called as C1 inhibitor) by limiting the actual time C1q gets to cleave C4 and C2 proteins;

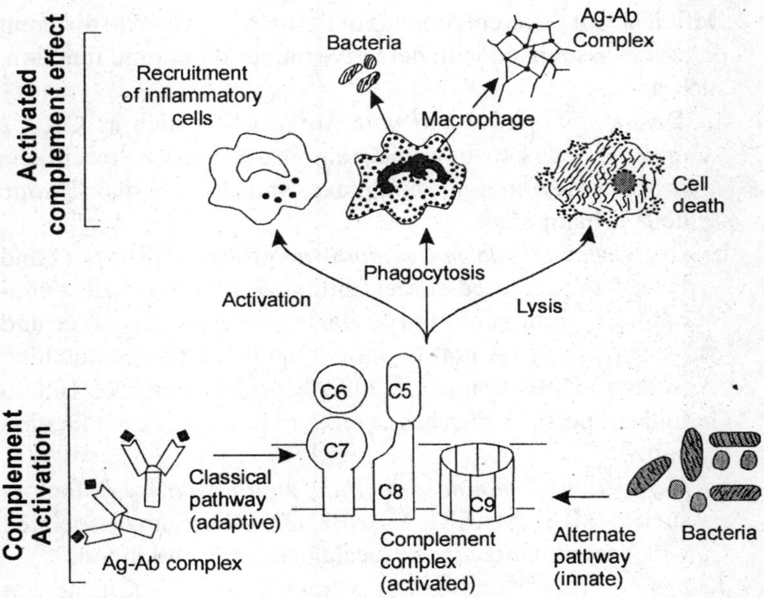

Figure 2.6: Effect of activated complement proteins

b. The *C4 binding protein* regulates the classical pathway of the fluid phase;

c. *Factor H* competes with factor B for binding with the factor C3b. If factor B wins, which would happen if bacterial surfaces have activated the complement pathway then the complete pathway is amplified. If factor H wins then the bound C3 factor to the H is catalyzed by factor I to form iC3b and C3dg and the complement activation in inhibited.

d. *Pronectin* or *CD59* protein inhibits the binding of C9 to the C5b,6,7 complex and therefore preventing its random insertion in the cell membrane.

Deficiency of Complement Proteins

- Defects in complement components are associated with susceptibility to many infections and accumulation of lethal immune complexes in the body.

- Deficiency of different proteins of the pathways lead to different disorders associated with defective humoral immune function, such as
  a. *Deficiency of classical pathway* proteins such as C1, C2 and C4 leads to immune complex disease wherein the processing of immune complexes and clearing of apoptotic cells is hampered.
  b. *Deficiency of alternative pathway* proteins, factors D and P lead to increased susceptibility to infection with extra-cellular pathogens, particularly pyogenic bacteria and *Neisseria* spp (A normal individual has a risk of catching *Neisseria* infection is 1/2,000,000 which increases 10,000 fold in a person which has a defect in the complement fixation pathway).
  c. *Deficiency of mannose-binding lecithin pathway* factors such as MBL, MASP1, MASP2, C2, C4 etc. are associated with bacterial infections especially in early childhood.
  d. *Defects in C3 convertase system* when C3 fails to get deposited, infection with *Neisseria spp.* and pyogenic bacteria is more probable. Certain times immune complex disorder is also generated.
  e. *Deficiency of MAC complex* proteins, *viz.* C5-C9 proteins lead to increased susceptibility to *Neisseria* infection.

Complement Fixation Test

- The test is based on the competition for complement, between various antigen-antibody complexes and the lytic system consisting the RBC-specific antibodies and RBC which, together with complement bring about the lysis of RBCs.
- The test consists of an indicator system composed of predetermined amount of sheep red blood cells (sRBC), rabbit antibodies to sRBC (also termed as hemolysin), and complement (C), which is generally supplied as guinea pig serum.
- The amounts of each reagent are predetermined in such a way that the introduction of complement, given at a slight deficiency, to sRBC-anti-sRBC complex (often termed as 'sensitized' RBC) results in almost complete (e.g. 95 %) lysis. The degree

of lysis can be determined spectrophotometrically by measuring the intensity of red color of hemoglobin released into the solution.

- Since the amount of complement is limiting, any loss or consumption of the complement would be reflected by a decrease in the extent of lysis. Such as loss occurs during preincubation of that fixed amount of complement with an antigen-antibody complex (not related to sRBC and anti-sRBC) that would result in the attachment of the complement to the antibody in this antigen-antibody complex.
- Subsequent introduction of sRBC-anti-sRBC in the complex does not result in the lysis of sRBC because the complex has been fixed or utilized by the first antigen-antibody system. The more complement is fixed by the first system, the more inhibition of lysis would be seen for the second sRBC system.
- The fixation of the complement by an antigen-antibody complex can be plotted as function of antigen concentration or a function of antibody concentration.

Table 2.3: The complement fixation test

Test system	*Order of component addition*			*Hemolysis*
	C	*sRBC*	*Anti – sRBC*	
Antigen X	+	+	+	Hemolysis
Antibody to X	+	+	+	Hemolysis
X–Anti X complex	+	+	+	No hemolysis
No test	+	+	+	Hemolysis

Chapter 3

Components of an Immune Response —Antigen and Antibody

An immune response involves two components, the cause or the invader and the response or neutralizer. These entities have been termed as '*antigens*' and '*antibodies*' in context of the immune system.

I. ANTIGEN

An immune response is generated in response to a 'non-self' molecule or antigen. Technically any molecule which is non-self should be termed as antigen, but certain features govern their antigenicity and their potential to generate systemic response. Such 'antigenic' features include:

1. **Source**, the self or non-self (foreign) dilemma. It is simple assumption that any '*foreign*' molecule/ entity is antigenic and would lead to generation of an immune reaction. Does it mean that any molecule or substance from one source or body would be antigenic in another body or person? In other words, can a protein from individual X generate an immune response in individual Y?

Immunologically, any molecule whose 'homologs' are present in the individual would fail to generate an immune response. The term 'homolog' refers to a chemically and structurally similar compound. Therefore, in this context, a protein from individual X would not generate an immune response in individual Y, but can generate a reaction in organism of different species like rat, sheep or horse. But, if the protein in question is a conserved protein and necessary for functioning in other animals as well, then it would either generate a weak response or fail to generate response, depending upon the degree of conservation between various homologs. Consequently, it is the degree of foreignness which decides degree of immunogenicity of the antigen. However, in exceptional conditions an individual mounts an immune response against his/ her own tissues. This condition is termed as autoimmunity (Chapter 8).

2. **Chemical nature and complexity,** the higher the complexity of an antigen, more the chances and strength of the immune response. It is best explained by the knowledge that infection by an organism like bacteria or protozoa generates a better immune response than a single protein. Proteins, by far are the best antigen, because of several layers of complexity associated with them which include their ability to multimerize or form complexes, their variable amino acid composition and 3-D structural variations, besides their potential in forming complex with carbohydrates and lipids. Keeping this complexity issue and their lineage in mind, various compounds can be arranged on scale in terms of their antigenicity,
   Proteins > Carbohydrates > Lipids > Small compounds
3. **Size or molecular weight,** similar to the complexity principle, the size of the antigen is directly proportional to its antigenicity. In general, compounds that have a molecular weight of less than 1,000 Da (e.g. drugs or hormones) are not immunogenic and those of molecular weight between 1,000 and 6,000 Da (e.g. hormones like insulin, etc.) may or may not be immunogenic and those with molecular weight greater than 6,000 Da are generally good immunogens.
   - Generally, for immunogenicity, the substances should have all the three mentioned features—it should be *foreign*; it

should be of *high molecular weight* and must possess a certain degree of *complexity*

- **Haptens** are low molecular weight compounds which are not immunogenic themselves but become immunogenic when complexed or conjugated with high molecular weight compounds. For example, DNP (dinitrophenazine) is not immunogenic but on coupling with tetanus toxin it becomes immunogenic.
- **Epitope** is the smallest entity of an antigen which is recognized as an antigen. In other words, it is the '*antigenic determinant*' region of an antigen.
- **Superantigens** are antigens which can lead to excessive activation of the cells of the immune system through non-specific binding to immune receptors, e.g. certain bacterial toxins (staphylococcal enterotoxins) and reteroviral proteins. Such antigens lead to excessive secretion of cytokines from the effector cells, which might lead to the development of toxin shock syndrome.

II. ANTIBODY

Antibodies or serum '*immunoglobulins*' is the term given to a group of serum molecules produced by the B-lymphocytes. They are essentially soluble and secreted form of B-cell receptors (BCR) and they are produced in large quantities to counter an invasion process by an antigen–hence the terminology '*antibody*'.

1. Structure of an Antibody Molecule

Since the antibody molecules are produced in large quantities by the B-cells without any manipulation, they have been studied extensively much before other insoluble cell receptors were analyzed. Detailed biochemical, physiological and genetic characterization of the antibody molecules revealed the following features:

- Each antibody molecule is composed of four chains-two identical ones called as *heavy chains* and other two identical ones as *light chains* based on their molecular weight or sizes. The individual chains are linked with each other through specific disulphide linkages. Heavy chains (H) of 53 kDa linked with each other form the central backbone of the antibody molecule with the light chain (L) of 22 kDa support the heavy chains from either side. For elucidation of this structure of antibody molecule Edelman and Porter were awarded the Noble Prize.

- The antigen recognizing region is composed of both heavy and light chains and is termed as '*Fab*' (fragment of antibody activity).
- The region which binds to various cells and activate various cells involved in neutralizing the antigen-antibody complex is termed as '*Fc*' region. It is also involved in anchoring of antibody molecules onto various cell surfaces.
- The variability of antigen recognition is determined by the '*variable*' region present in both the heavy and light chains.
- The non-variable regions of the heavy and light chains is called as the '*constant*' regions.
- Light chains have two genetically variable types – kappa (κ) and lambda (λ), whereas heavy chains are of five types, classified on the basis of type of antibody molecule.
- Detailed structural features of an antibody molecule revealed the following features:
  - Interchain disulphide bonds hold together the H and L-chains.
  - Intrachain disulphide bonds provide the characteristic 'loop' fold of the antibody chains. Each loop consists of 100-110 amino acids and is involved in formation of a compact globular structure called as '*globular domain*'. Two such domains are present in light chains and four in heavy chains. Each constant domain is designated by a letter that indicates its presence on heavy chain followed by a number, e.g. the second domain in heavy chain is designated as C_H1.
  - In heavy chains of immunoglobulins, a '*hinge region*' is present between the domain 2 and 3 (C_H1 and C_H2), which is rich in cysteine and proline residues. This region provides flexibility to the antigen-binding two arms of the Y-shaped Fab regions.

– Proteolytic cleavage of the antibody molecule was the first indirect proof about the structure function aspects of the antibody molecule. Enzyme papain cleaves at the hinge region generating 1 Fc and 2 Fab fragments. The Fab region can bind to the antigen and Fc region can be crystallized. Compared to this enzyme pepsin cleaves the antibody into 1 discrete $F(ab)_2$ region which binds to antigen with higher affinity, is of larger size as well and many smaller degradative byproducts of the Fc region. These experiments provide support to the structural idea that antigen-binding region (Fab) is dimeric entity and cell-activating entity Fc region is common to both the Fab region (Fig. 3.2).

2. Types of Antibody Molecules

Depending on the structure, source, polymorphism and other effector functions mediated by them, the antibodies have been classified in following types:

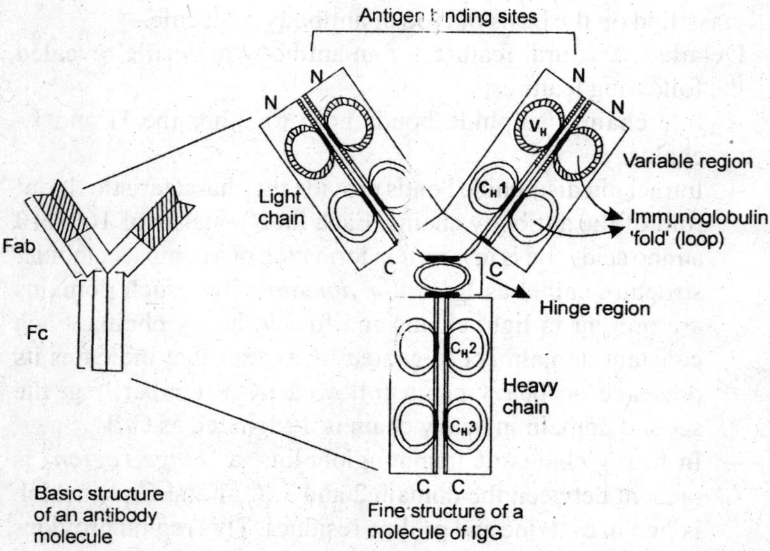

Figure 3.1: Structure of an antibody molecule.

Table 3.1: Types of immunoglobulin molecules and their discriminating features

Feature	*IgG*	*IgA*	*IgM*	*IgD*	*IgE*
Nature	Monomer	Dimer	Pentamer	Monomer	Monomer
Mol. Wt. (kDa)	150,000	160,000 for monomer	900,000	180,000	200,000
Additional proteins	None	J or T or S chains	J chain	None	None
Source	Serum	Secretions	Intravas-cular	On cell surface	Mast cells, basophils
Serum conc. (mg/ml)	12	1.8	1	0 – 0.04	0.00002
Percentage of IgG	80	13	6	0.2	0.002
Half-life (days)	23	5.5	5	2.8	2.0
Heavy chain	γ	α	μ	δ	ε
Placental passage	++	–	–	–	–
Presence in secretions	–	+	–	–	–
Complement activation	+	–	+++	–	–
Effector functions	Ag neutra-lization		Primary antibody		
Antibacterial activity	+++	++	+++	–	–
Antitoxin activity	+++	–	–	–	–
Allergic activity	–	–	–	–	++
Other nome-nclature	Common	Secretory	Pentamer	Memory	Allergic or reaginic

- **Paratope** is the epitope binding site of an antibody molecule. These regions are essentially formed by the variable CDR regions.
- **Idiotope** is the antigenic determinant (epitope) region of an antibody molecule which can bind to the paratopes of other antibodies. This region is essentially present in the variable regions of the antibody molecule.

3. Monoclonal Antibodies

Encounter with an antigen in the body leads to the development of a generalized immune response to the entire antigen and leads to generation of antibody response to all the epitopes of an antigen.

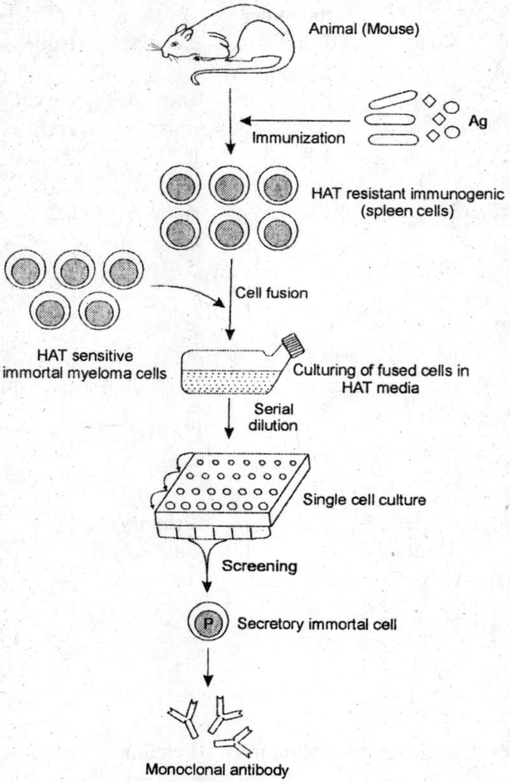

Figure 3.2: Monoclonal antibody production

This leads to the generation of the antibodies to various antigenic determinants and hence the immune response is a random mix of antibodies. However, antibodies of a single specificity are highly desired for many applications including diagnostic tests, immunotherapy, etc. Such single specificity antibodies are called as '*monoclonal antibodies*' and they are essentially generated by specialized *in vitro* cell fusion protocols developed by Kohler and Milstein in the 1970s (Fig. 3.2).

The method essentially involves following steps:

1. Generation of antibody response in an animal using purified antigen and isolation of antibody producing lymphoid cells from spleen of immunized animal.
2. The antibody-secreting lymphoid cells are then fused with 'immortal' (malignant) cells leading to the formation of immortal antibody producing B-cells (product of cell fusion).
3. Such immortal cells are diluted to obtain single immortal cell, which are then cultivated to obtain a single population of secretory cells called as "pure cell line".
4. The individual secretory cell population are then analyzed secreted antibodies in terms of their antigen binding capabilities.

Since, such antibody producing immortal cells are essentially derived from a single antibody-secretory cell, the antibodies they produce are termed '*monoclonal antibodies*'.

4. Antigen–Antibody Interaction

- The binding of the Ag-Ab complex can be disrupted by high salt concentrations, extremes of pH, detergents and even by competition with pure antigen itself indicating that the interactions are necessarily reversible non–covalent.
- Ag-Ab interactions involve a number of forces, which include:
  a. Electrostatic forces
  b. Hydrogen bonds
  c. Van der waals forces
  d. Hydrophobic forces

The contribution of each of these forces in the overall interaction depends upon particular Ag–Ab complex.

5. Effector Functions of Antibodies

Though primary function of an antibody molecule is to neutralize antigen, it can seldom do this on its own and the actual process of antigen neutralization involves many downstream processes which are initiated after the antigen-antibody complex is formed. These processes include:

a. Macrophage recruitment, activation and antigen processing
b. Complement activation by classical pathway.
c. Antibody dependent cell cytotoxicity
d. Activation of effector functions through Fc receptor binding
e. Hypersensitivity response through mast cell degranulation and accumulation of Ag-Ab complex.

Chapter 4

Immune Recognition

It is the nature of the antigen which decides the type of immune response which will be mounted against it. Essentially it involves the following processes, (a) *antigen entry*, (b) *antigen recognition and processing*, (c) *activation of immune cells by the processed antigen* and (d) *destruction and removal of the antigen*. Besides a number of proteins which contribute to these processes, three types of cells are central to these responses.

ANTIGEN PRESENTING CELLS (APCs)

- A number of cells can serve as antigen processing cells depending on their ability to recognize, engulf and process antigens. Such cells include macrophages, dendritic cells, Kupffer cells, microglial cells, etc. and includes B-cells as well which engulf Ag in association with surface Ig.
- *Macrophages* are primary immune cells which develop from monocytes which first encounters the antigen. These cells serve multiple functions in the host immune system which includes
  a. Antigen uptake, processing and presentation, acting as an antigen presenting cell (APC).
  b. Opsonization and phagocytosis function of the macrophages is decided by certain proteins of the microbes and other activates proteins and cytokines from the host.

Table 4.1: Properties of various antigen presenting cells

Feature	*Antigen presenting cell type*		
	Dendritic cell	*Macrophage*	*B-cell*
Antigen uptake	By macropino-cytosis and phagocytosis	By phagocytosis	Through antigen – specific receptor (surface antibody)
MHC expression	Low in tissue localized cells. High in lymphoid tissue localized cells	Low and inducible by bacteria and cytokines	Constitutive expression which gets induced after activation
Co-stimulator delivery	Constitutive expression by mature non-phagocytic cells	Low but inducible	Low but inducible
Antigens presented	Peptides Viral antigens Allergens	Particulate antigens Intracellular and extracellular pathogens	Soluble antigens Toxins Viruses
Localization	Lymphoid tissue Connective tissue Epithelia	Lymphoid tissue Connective tissue Body cavities	Lymphoid tissue Peripheral blood

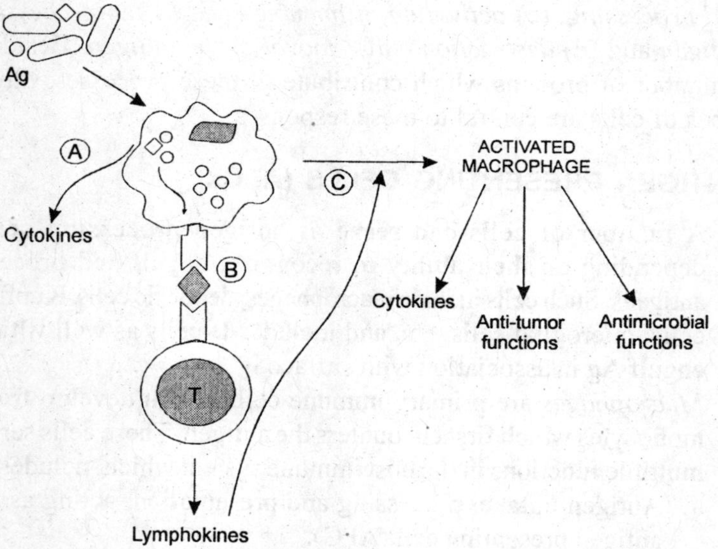

Figure 4.1: Central role of macrophages (A) Initial defence (phagocytosis) (B) Antigen processing and presentation (C) Effector activities

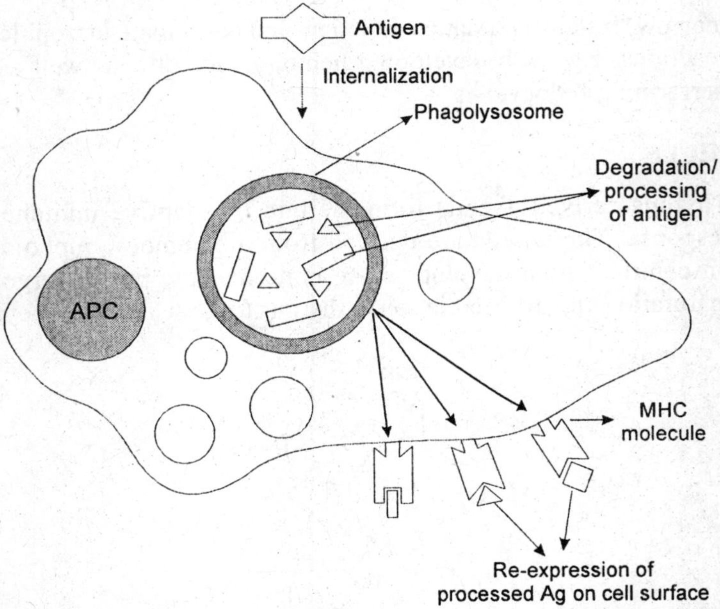

Figure 4.2: Antigen presenting cells as central component to CMI

- Immunologically primed macrophages differ from resident macrophages. Monocyte recruitment is enhanced and yields macrophages with proinflammatory and cytotoxic properties. Activation by cytokines enhances expression of MHC class II and the complement receptor CR3. Phagocytosis and the production of proinflammatory mediators and cytotoxic products are increased. By contrast, resident macrophages (e.g. in bone

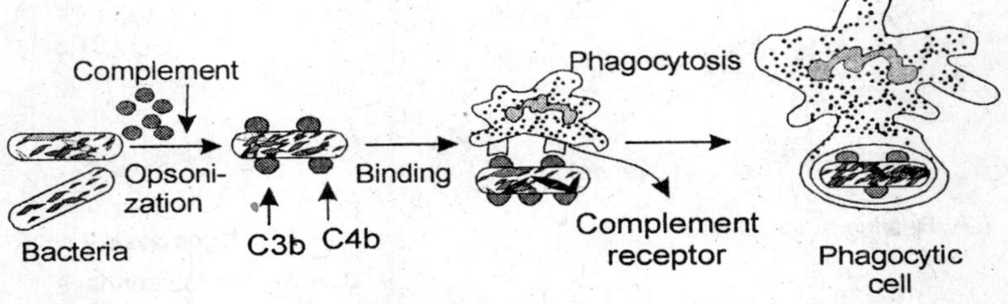

Figure 4.3: Opsonization and phagocytosis by macrophages

marrow) lack inflammatory functions but participate in trophic reactions, e.g. with developing hemopoietic cells, as well as performing endocytosis.

T-CELLS

- Thymus-derived T-cells form the hub of adaptive immune response. These cells are derived from a common lymphoid progenitor which develop in the bone marrow but undergo maturation and differentiation in thymus to form T-cells. They

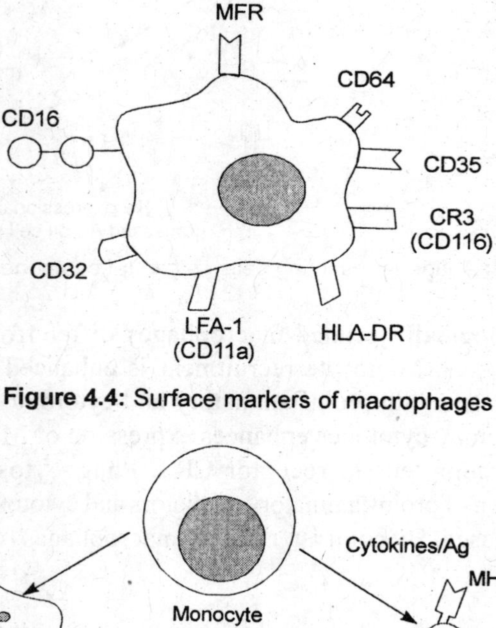

Figure 4.4: Surface markers of macrophages

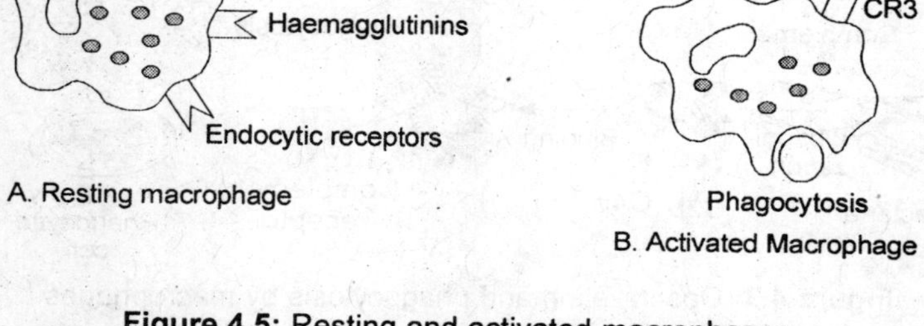

Figure 4.5: Resting and activated macrophages

differentiate in thymus from as $CD4^+$ $CD8^+$ (α:β T-cell progenitor) cells to $CD4^+$ $CD8^-$ (T_H) and $CD4^-$ $CD8^+$ (T_C) cells. Discrimination of self-protein and non-self protein recognition amongst T-cell takes place in thymus only. The cells which detect self antigens in association with MHC are deleted by a process termed as '*clonal deletion*'. Approximately 1–2 % of total T-cell population present in the thymus enters the peripheral organs and rest die by apoptosis.

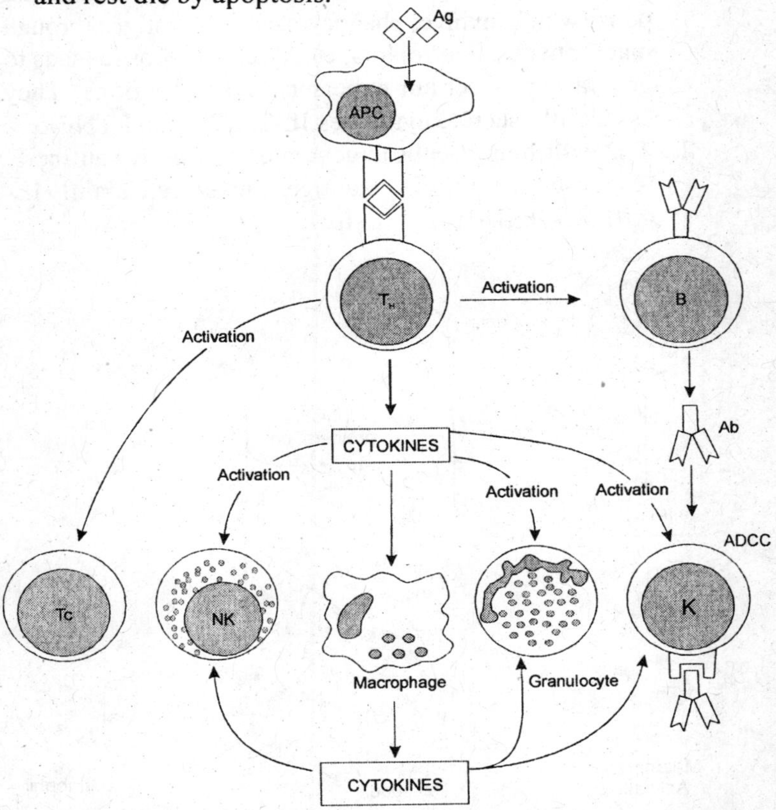

Figure 4.6: Central role of T_H-cells in cell-mediated immunity and communication networks and cytokines

- These are $CD2^+$ $CD3^+$ cells and are essentially of two sub-types–T_H and T_C depending on the nature of antigen presentation, which ultimately decides the outcome of immune response.

a. **T_H cells**–Termed as T-helper cells as they are essentially involved in helping the antibody producing B-cells or macrophages in mounting an effective antigen-clearing immune response. These cells are $CD4^+$ $CD8^-$ cells and recognize antigen presented to them with MHC-II only. Depending on the effector cells they help, they are further categorized in 2 classes – T_H1 and T_H2 cells.

1. **T_H1 cells** help to generate an inflammatory immune response which involves phagocytosis of the antigen through macrophages, neutrophils, etc. Such a response leads to generation of certain hypersensitivity reactions. They essentially secrete cytokines IL-2, IFN-γ and TNF-α.
2. **T_H2 cells** help B-cells to generate an effective antibody response for neutralizing antigen and secrete mainly IL-4,IL-5,IL-6,IL-10 and IL-13.

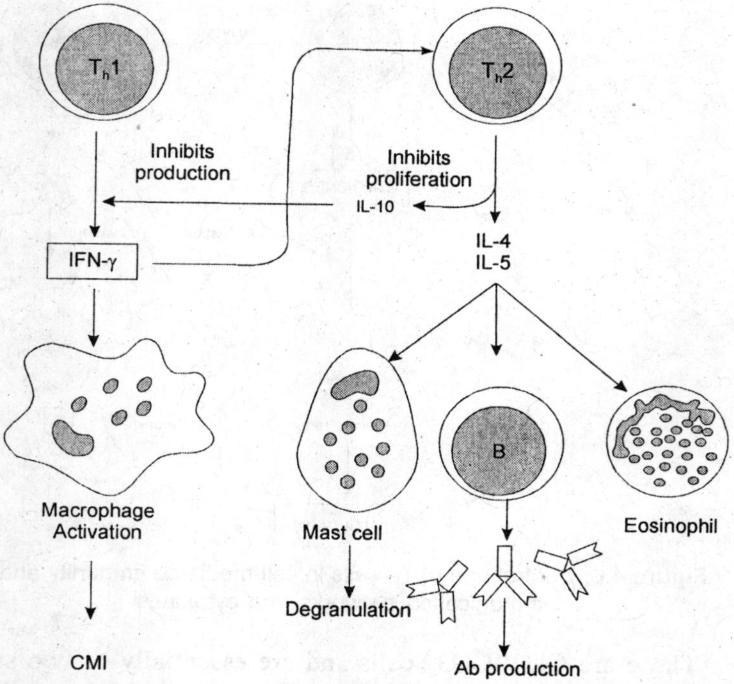

Figure 4.7: Selection of T_H1 and T_H2 responses and their effector mechanisms

b. **T_C cells**–Cytotoxic T-cells as they can neutralize the host cells infected with antigen (e.g. viruses) by destroying them through various processes such as perforin activation. The recognize antigen presented to them by APC in association with MHC-I. These are $CD8^+$ $CD4^-$ cells.

- These cells recognize antigen presented to them by only an antigen presenting cell (APC) and cannot interact with antigen alone. Immune response only in conjunction with MHC (major histocompatibility complex).

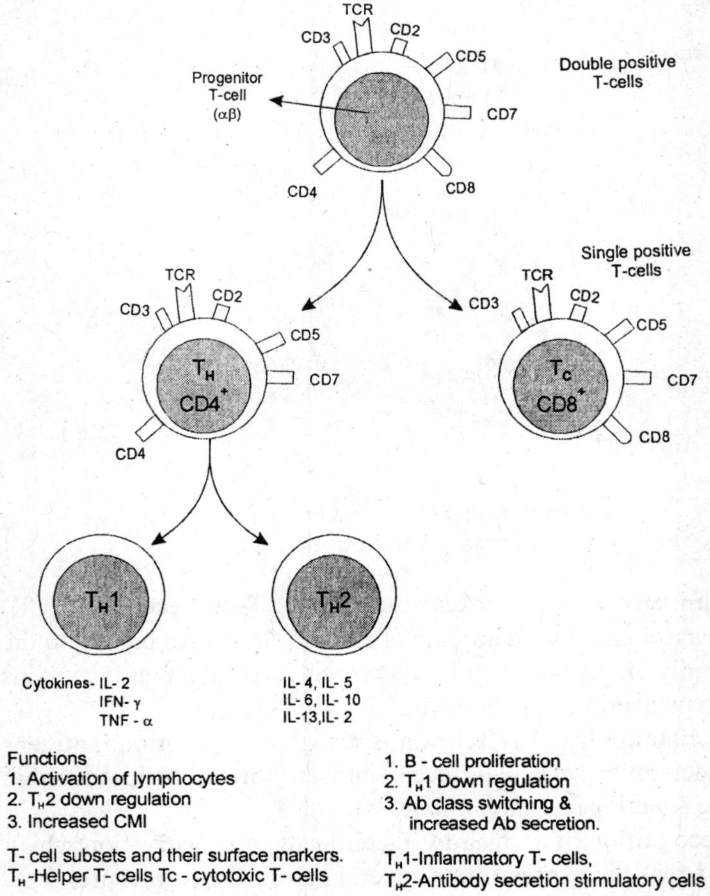

Figure 4.8: Subtypes of T-cells and their immune responses.

- Presentation of antigen processed by APCs in association of MHC complexes also requires co-stimulatory signals from the APC such as interaction between B7 receptor and CD28 marker without which the T-cell activation fails to take place. The B7 receptor is located on the APC and the corresponding receptor CD28 on T-cell. Both CD28 and B7 proteins are members of immunoglobulin superfamily. B7 is a homodimer, each of whose chain has a immunoglobulin V-like domain and one C-like domain. CD28 is a disulphide-linked homodimer in which each chain has one V-like domain.

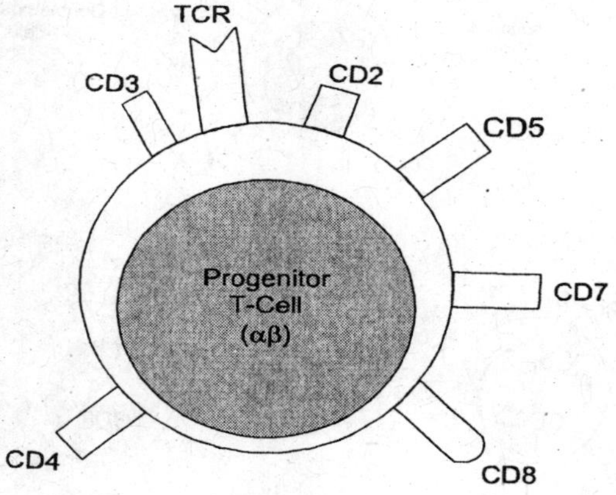

Figure 4.9: Surface markers of a progenitor αβ T- cells (double-positive cell)

- Antigen recognition takes place through T-cell receptors (TCR) in association with appropriate MHC. TCR also belong to the family of immunoglobulin superfamily of proteins as it contains a typical immunoglobulin fold.
- Variability in the TCR towards recognition of various antigens is determined at genetic levels similar to variability introduced in the B-cell receptors (antibodies).
- Recognition of antigen by T-cell leads to its activation which changes the expression of several cell surface molecules.

Table 4.2: Change in cell-surface molecules of a T_H cell on activation

Cell-surface marker	*Status of the marker in T_H cell*	
	Resting cell	*Activated cell*
L – selectin	+	-
VLA-4	-	+
LFA-1	+	++
CD2	+	++
CD4	+	+
TCR	+	+
CD44	+	++
CD45RA	+	-
CD45RO	-	+

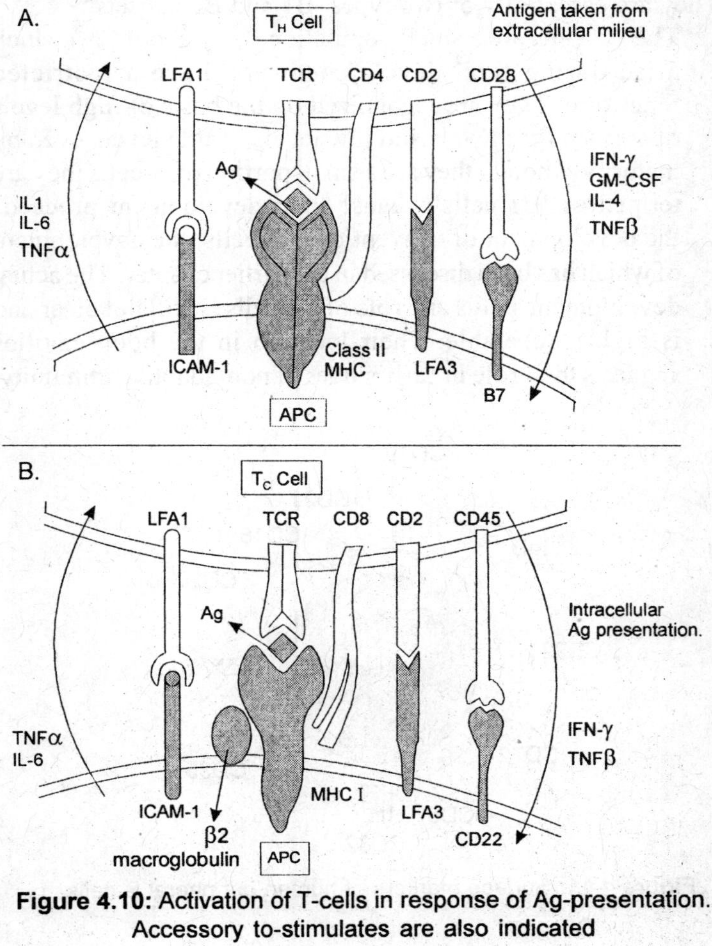

Figure 4.10: Activation of T-cells in response of Ag-presentation. Accessory to-stimulates are also indicated

B-CELLS

- Bone-marrow derived cells are essentially antibody-producing $CD19^{+}CD22^{+}$ cells which differentiate into antibody producing '*plasma cells*' or antigen–specificity remembering '*memory – cells*' in response to an encounter with antigen, which is detected though IgD molecules expressed on its surface.
- Its recognition of antigen does not involve any direct helper molecule like T0-cells but the process of differentiation is dependent on T_H2 cells.
- They are essentially of two types–B1 and B2 subsets.
  1. The **B1 cells** are a small population (only about 5%) which arise during fetal development and have a restricted repertoire. They are recognized on the basis of high levels of surface IgM levels and low levels of IgD levels even on maturity. Though they are a small portion of B-cells they are termed as 'B1'cells because their development proceeds the development of conventional B-cells, the development of which has been discussed in the earlier chapter. The actual development status and role of B1 cells is still not clear and is highly debatable. Their location in the body cavities suggests their role in early stages of non-adaptive immunity.

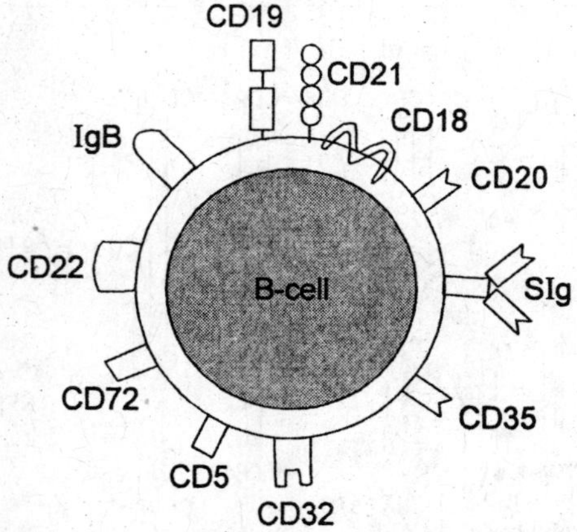

Figure 4.11: Surface markers of human peripheral B-cells

2. The **B2 cells** are the conventional B-cells which have a diverse repertoire and express higher levels of surface IgD on maturity.

- The genetic variability of B-cells receptor which is involved in initial identification and further neutralization of antigens is pre-determined by the genetic variability of the BCR. The variability of the BCR is governed by multiple processes which includes:

i. *Presence of multiple genes for each chain:* different genes code for the variable and constant regions of the heavy (H) and light (L) chains.

ii. *Genetic recombination of various genes:* Any of the many different variable region genes can be linked to a single constant region gene to form many permutations of the genes, thus conserving DNA.

iii. *Joining segment and diversity segment:* Joining segment is the additional gene sequence required during the formation of L chain. It joins the V_L region gene to the C_L region gene and the diversity segment similarly joins the V_H gene to the J gene. These genes are then fused with the C_H gene, during the formation of the H-chain.

iv. *H-chain class switching:* T-cell cytokines (IL-4, IL-13, IFN-γ, TGF-β) mediate the switching from μ to δ to $\gamma3,\gamma1,\alpha1,\gamma2,\gamma4$ and $\alpha2$ through later rearrangement of the class genes in the C_H region.

v. *somatic hypermutation*: Mutational hotspots in the genes leads to further variability.

- These factors along with random selection of V, D, J genes by each B-cell and allelic exclusion of one of the two parallel alleles by a single B-cell resulting in a single H-chain isotype and L-chain subtype receptor, ensure generation of a huge repertoire of antigen-recognition BCR on the B-cells.
- Once these variable BCRs are generated, their further selection and proliferation of these naïve B-cells take place via an antigen-dependent process termed as clonal-selection. This process leads to the generation of antibody-secreting B-cell derivative 'plasma cells' and non-secretory but activated '*memory cells*' which

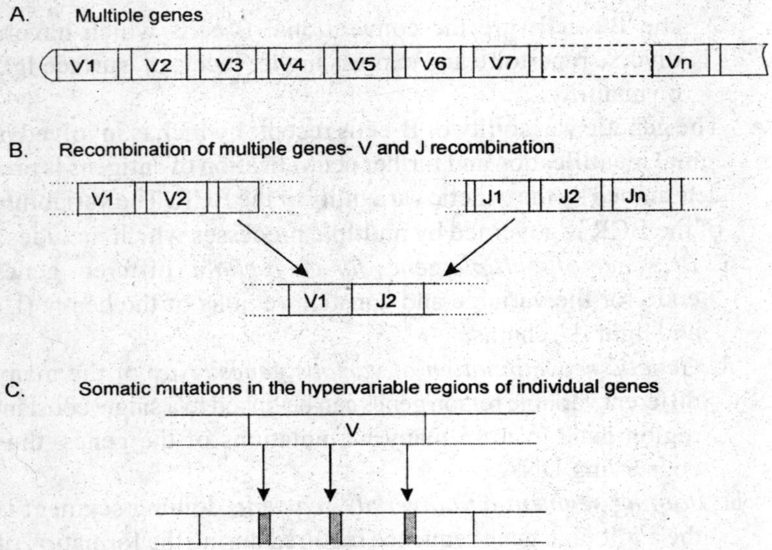

Figure 4.12: Variability in the immunoglobulin molecules

can rapidly differentiate into plasma cells in future encounters with the antigen and can mount a stronger immune response.

- The formation and prolonged life cycle of the memory-cells is the principle behind vaccination. In the initial dose of the vaccine, the naïve B-cell differentiates into small population of antibody secreting plasma cells and memory cells hence a very low titer of antibodies is obtained. During the next dose of the vaccine the memory cells rapidly proliferate on antigen encountering to form a large population of antibody-secreting plasma cells; hence a higher titer of antibodies is obtained. During subsequent challenges the countering time from the memory cells decreases and the net proliferation and antibody response also increases.

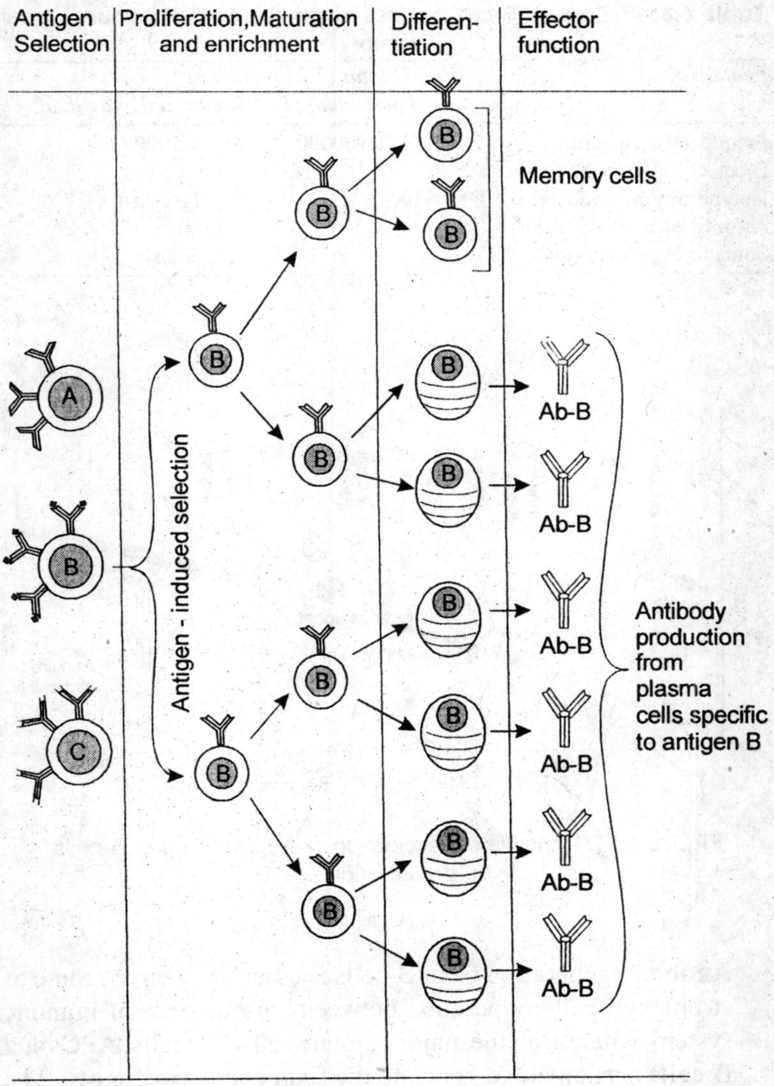

Figure 4.13: Clonal selection theory and selection of naïve B-cells into plasma cells

Table 4.3: Analysis of B-cell features as an outcome of immunological memory

Feature of B-cell	*Status of the feature in*	
	Unimmunized individual	*Immunized individual*
Frequency of specific B-cells	1:10000 – 1:100000	1:1000
Isotype of Ab produced	IgM > IgG	IgG, IgA
Affinity of antibody	Low	High
Somatic hypermutation	Low	High

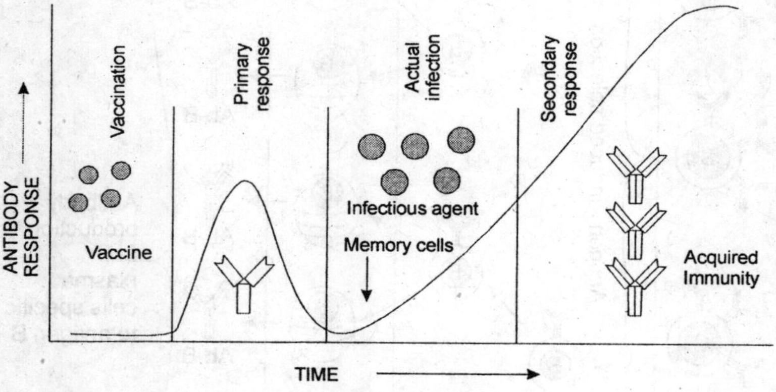

Figure 4.14: Principle of vaccination in the backdrop of B-cells proliferation.

- Antibody-generation from B-cells is essentially an outcome of strong cell-cell cooperation between various cells of immune system, wherein all the major immune cells—T-cells, APCs and B-cells participate to generate the final countering entity. The participation of cells is through intense communication between all cells by the cytokine networks.

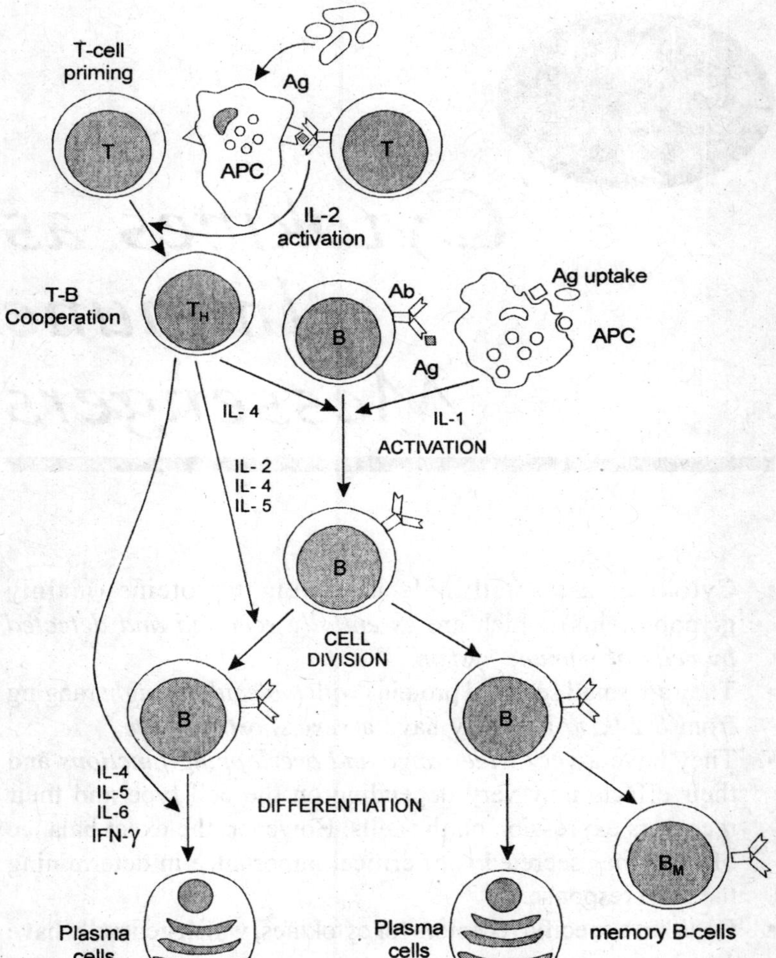

Figure 4.15: B cell activation, development and T-cell cooperation in Ab-production

Chapter 5

Cytokines as Immune Messengers

- Cytokines are small molecular weight proteins (mainly glycoproteins) which are *essentially secreted and detected by cells of immune system.*
- They are small secreted proteins with *molecular weight* ranging from *8-24kDa* and they have a *very short half-life.*
- They have a very *wide range and overlapping functions* and their effects may vary depending on the cell type and their receptors expression on the cells. However, the exact balance of cytokines secreted is of critical importance in determining the final response.
- Cells have specific receptors for cytokines, which generally have 1 to 3 subunits.
- The multi-faceted effects of cytokines include:
  a. Activation/ inhibition/ potentiation/ dimunition of numerous functions of leukocytes especially in immune responses and inflammation, e.g. chemotaxis.
  b. Antiviral responses which can be induced in many cell types particularly by interferons.
  c. Induction of apoptosis of infected cells especially by TNF-β.

d. Growth factor activities on hematopoietic ells, fibroblasts, endothelial cells, etc.

Table 5.1: Functions of some-well defined T-cell cytokines

Cytokines	*T-cell source*	*Functions*
IL-2	T_H0, T_H1 and CTL	Growth of T-cells, NK cells, stimulation of B-cells and J-chain synthesis
IFN-g	T_H1 and CTL	Activation of macrophages, increase in expression of class I and class II MHC, inhibits T_H2 cell growth, activation of NK cells
TNF-b	T_H1 and some CTL	Activated macrophages, induced NO production by them. Kills T-cells and activates neutrophils besides killing of tumor cells and fibroblasts
IL-4	T_H2	Induces growth and survival of T- cells; activates B-cells and induces class II MHC expression on them; inhibits macrophage activation and increases growth of mast cells
IL-5	T_H2	Increases eosinophil growth and differentiation and leads to differentiation of IgA synthesis in B-cells
IL-10	T_H2	Inhibits T_H1 cells; inhibits cytokine release from macrophages; co-stimulates mast cell growth
IL-3	T_H1, T_H2 and some CTL	Serves as growth factor for progenitor hemato-poietic cells (acts as multi–CSF)
TNF-a	T_H1, some T_H2 and some CTL	Activated macrophages, induced NO production by them.
GM-CSF	T_H1, some T_H2 and some CTL	Increases production of granulocytes, macrophages and dendritic cells from hematopoietic cells; inhibits growth of T-cells; causes activation of macrophages
TGF-b	CD4 cells	Inhibits activation of macrophages; activates neutro-phils; inhibits growth of B-cells and IgA switching.

- The nomenclature of cytokines partly reflects their first-described function and also the order of their discovery. There is no single unified nomenclature, and individual cytokines may belong to two groups, e.g. the chemokine interleukin-8 (IL-8). Although they are generally grouped as family, the exact notion of 'family' is more functional rather than structural, as most of these proteins are not chemically related at all.

- *Types of cytokines:*
  1. Interleukins – IL-1 to IL-14 (and beyond)
  2. Interferons α, β and γ - IFN
  3. Tumor necrosis factors α and β - TNF
  4. Growth factors, EGF, NGF – GF
  5. Colony stimulating factors – GM, M, G - CSF
  4. Chemokines and chemotactic factors MIP -1α and β, MCP, RANTES, etc.

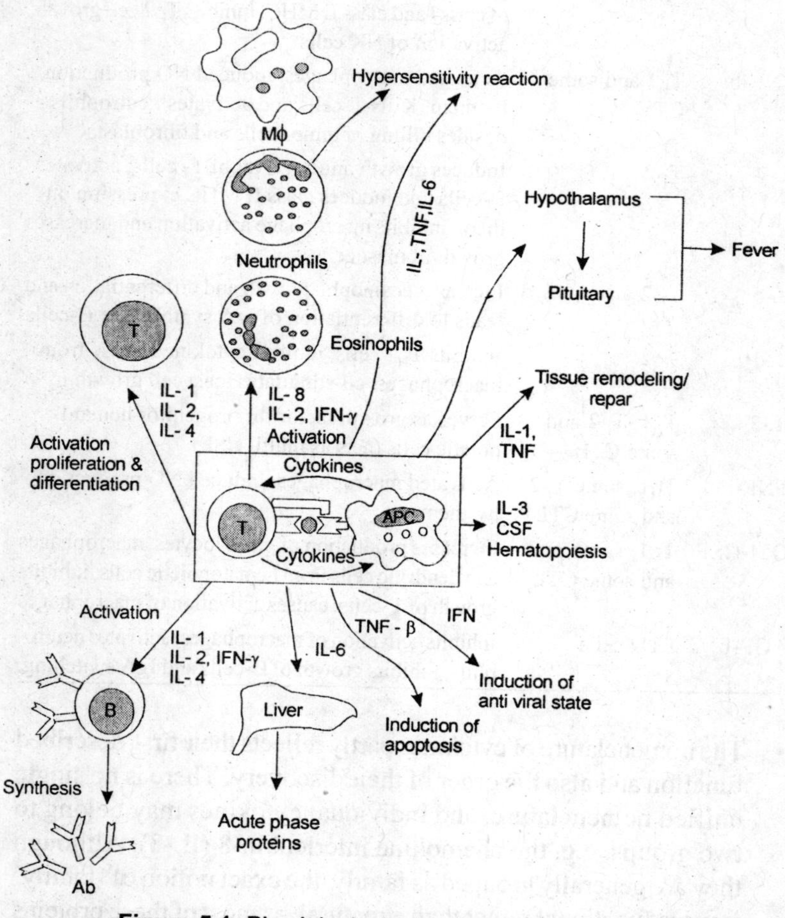

Figure 5.1: Physiological role of cytokine network (cytokine as communication link)

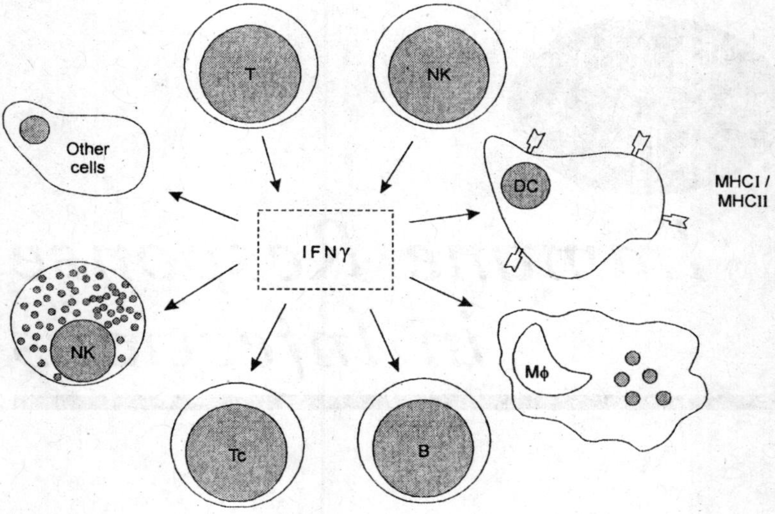

Figure 5.2: Effects of IL-1 and IL-2

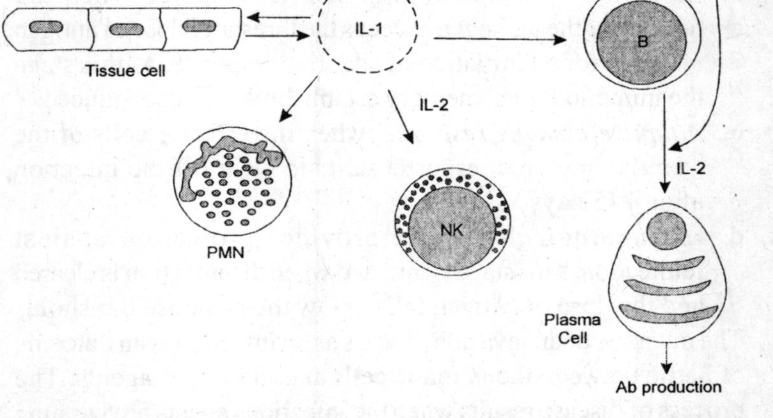

Figure 5.3: Action of IL-1 cytokine and its relation with IL-2 cytokine in activities some central immune reactions including Ab-production

Chapter 6

Immune Response in Infections

- Immune response to various infective organisms depends essentially on the nature of the pathogen.
- Irrespective of the nature of the pathogen or the infectious agent, a typical acute infection follows a well-defined course, which includes:
  a. *Establishment of infection*, wherein the level of the infectious agent increases as it undergoes replication
  b. *Induction of adaptive response* takes place when the number of the pathogen exceeds the threshold dose of antigen required for an initiation of adaptive response. At this stage the immunological memory establishment is also induced.
  c. *Adaptive immune response*, when the effector cells of the adaptive immune response starts to clear off the infection after 4 -5 days.
  d. *Immunological memory* provides protection against reinfection. This stage is initiated when the infection is cleared and the dose of antigen falls below the response threshold.
- The outcome of an invasion process as an infection is an outcome of battle between the immune cells and infectious agents. The process of disease results when the infectious agents are winning and treatment results when the immune system is winning.

- To evade the surveillance of the immune system, the pathogens constantly develop newer means and methods. Some of the well-established methods of evasion are:
  a. *antigenic variation*, term used to describe the change in the surface antigens of the pathogen. This essentially takes place by three processes
- Existance of wide variety of antigenic types of the pathogen. For example, *Streptococcus pneumoniae* which causes bacterial pneumonia exists in at least 84 different '*serotypes*' with each type differing from the previous on basis of the structure of its polysaccharide capsule.
- Evolution of antigenic types by antigenic drift or antigenic shift mechanisms as it happens in the case of influenza virus. Such process involves either modification in the surface proteins by smaller point mutations (leading to *antigenic drift*) or large scale genetic rearrangement of the surface receptor proteins (leading to *antigenic shift*). These changes in the surface molecules require mounting of fresh immune response and are poorly recognized by earlier antibodies.
- Programmed rearrangement of the DNA in the pathogen leads to variations in the surface antigens of the pathogen. Example of such variations includes variation in surface antigen of trypanosome, the causative pathogen of African trypanosomes.
  b. *Persistance*, which essentially involves *in vivo* maintenance of the pathogen in non-replicative form till the immunity wanes. Such processes are very effective mode of circumventing for intracellular pathogens like Herpes virus, Epstein-barr virus and even bacteria like *Mycobacterium tuberculosis* as their active replicating forms are easily countered by immune cells.

I. Immunity to Bacteria–Activation of T_H Cells

- A pathogen which is large and which can be detected by the immune system as an antigen generally gives rise to a strong B-cell response coupled with complement mediated neutralization of the pathogen, e.g. bacteria.
- Majority of the bacterial infections are tackled at the first line of defense, the barriers of the body. Most of the infections are limited at these entry points itself.

- If all the bacteria penetrate the first line of defense and enter tissues, they are initially combated by components of innate immunity without involving the cellular T- and B-cell components. Such processes include:
  a. Activation of complement pathway followed by anaphylotoxic effects of C3a and C5a proteins leading to mast cells degranulation which leads to increased vascular permeability, activation and recruitment of macrophages.
  b. Activation of TNF-mediated phagocytic pathways through C-reactive proteins and mannan-binding proteins present in the bacterial cell wall.
  c. Increased cell and fibrin adhesion to the endothelial cells mediated by secretion of TNF and IL-1 from phagocytic cells.
- Once bacterium is phagocytized, it is processed and presented to T_H cells to elicit a secondary immune response by activating B-cells to produce neutralizing antibodies through the T_H2 pathway.
- The antibacterium antibodies also have a multifaceted antibacterial effect, such as
  a. Antibodies to fimbriae, lipoteichoic acid and some capsules block attachment of the bacterium to the host cells.
  b. Antibodies can directly block many bacterial surface proteins which might be involved in 'sensing' or 'picking' molecules from surrounding milieu and transport them across membrane, e.g. for iron chelating compounds.
  c. Antibodies can serve as opsonins via Fc receptors.
  d. Immunorepellent molecules present on the bacterial surface which interfere with the phagocytosis can be effectively neutralized by antibodies.
  e. The bacterial toxins or enzymes which can elicit the toxic effect of the bacterial infection can also be effectively neutralized by the antibodies, e.g. diphtheria toxin.

II. Immunity to Viruses–Activation of the T_C cells

- Viruses as a pathogen must enter a host cell to proliferate and cause disease. The spectrum of disease caused by them is as variable as their genetic make-up, but there exits no correlation between the two.

- The illness or disease caused by them can be acute, recurrent, latent or dormant and might be in the subclinical stage only. Hence, the immune response generated against them is equally variable.
- The adaptive cell-mediated immune response depends on the recognition of specific antigens on the virus and virally-infected cells. Since antibodies can neutralize only the extracellular viruses, their action is largely limited due to presence of only a small population of extracellular virions in the host. Though an antibody-response is mounted against the virions, their effects are limited only to the following:
  a. Blocking of critical adhesion and effector sites of the virion,
  b. Lysis of the virion through the complement activated pathways and
  c. Activation of phagocytosis by forming an Ag-Ab complex.
- The cell-mediated immune reactions, directed though Tc cells are hence more effective in combating the virally infected cells.
- The major neutralizing effect against viruses is through interferons, which exert its effects through many pathways:
  a. Increased expression of class I and class II MHC facilitating recognition of viral antigens by the immune system.
  b. Activation of NK and macrophages which is capable of destroying virally-infected cells.
  c. Direct inhibition of viral replication by binding to IFN receptors on the neighboring cells, which induces synthesis of antiviral proteins such as a protein kinase and 2', 5' adenyl synthetase which leads to destruction of double-stranded RNA (the genetic material of most of the viruses).

III. Immunity to Fungi

- Precise mechanisms involved in fugal immunity are not known, but are thought to be similar to bacterial infections.

Types of Fungal Infection

- The fungal infections essentially fall into four categories

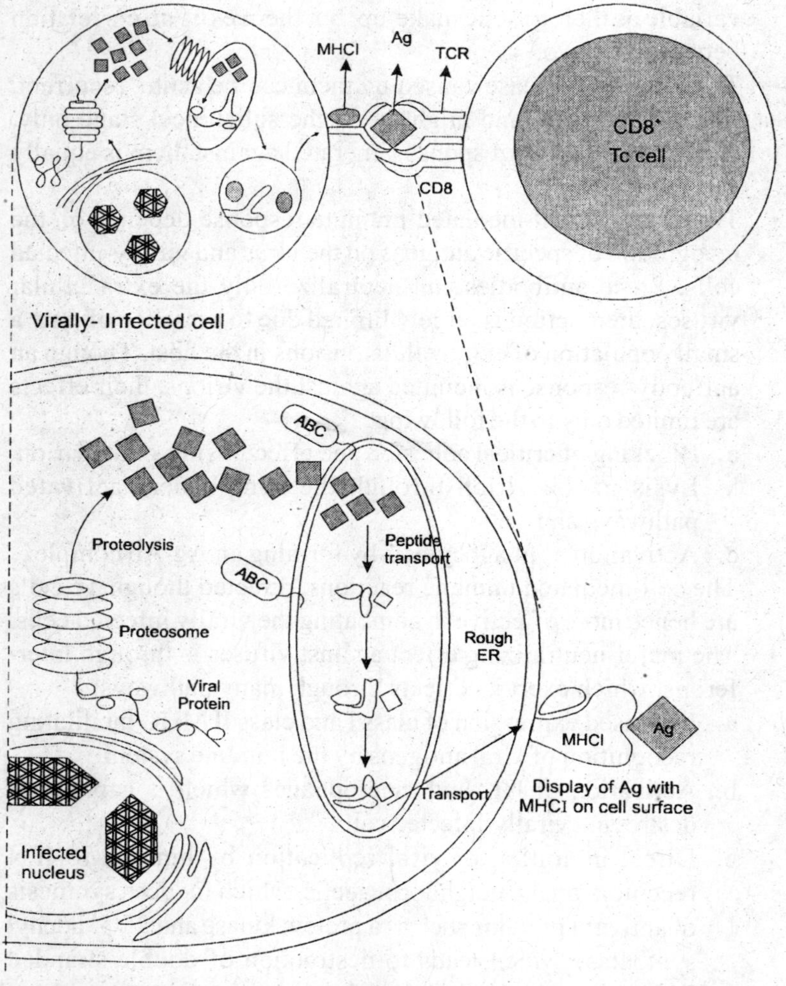

Figure 6.1: Antigen presentation of a virally-infected cell to T_C cell.

1. *Superficial mycoses* Caused by fungi known as dermatiphytes and the infections are restricted to non-living keratinized components such as skin, hair and nails.
2. *Subcutaneous mycoses* Caused by saprophytic fungi which causes chronic nodules or ulcers in subcutaneous tissues following trauma. For example, mycetoma, sprotrichosis, etc.

3. *Respiratory mycoses* Caused by soil saprophytes causing clinical or acute lung infections or granulomatous lesions.
4. *Candidiasis* Caused by a ubiquitous commensal *Candida albicans* causing infections of skin and mucous membranes.

Resistance and Protection

- Cutaneous fungi are generally self-limiting and recovery is associated with development of resistance.
- Resistance develops after failure of development of delayed-type hypersensitivity response which is generally mounted against fungal antigens.
- Infections by *Candida* are predominant in patients suffering from immunodeficiency disorders or in patients undergoing treatment with immunosuppressive drugs implying that immune system is involved in confining the fungus to its normal commensal sites in the body.
- There is also evidence for neutrophil polymorph involvement in immunity to some respiratory mycoses such as mucormycosis.
- It is also possible that the cationic proteins (defensins) produced by the phagocytes are important for protection from the fungi.

IV. Immunity of Protozoa and Worms

- Parasitic infections typically stimulate a number of immunological defense mechanisms, both antibody-mediated and cell-mediated, with the actual response depending upon the stage and cause of infection.
- Parasitic infections are caused by either protozoa or worms.
  a. Protozoa infect gut (*African trypansomes*), erythrocytes (*Plasmodium spp*), macrophages (*Leishmania spp.*), spleen, liver or muscle (*Trypanosoma cruzi*).
  b. Worms invade gut (tapeworms and hookworms), blood vessels (schistostomoses) and lymphatics (filarial worms).
- The parasities which infect human are simply the largest of all invaders. The large size of the pathogen also predispose them to stronger immune reaction as they express more of surface antigens.

- Though parasites might initiate a stronger immune response, they have evolved many different ways of evading them, which includes:
  - Intracellular localization inside the immune cells
  - Generation of antigenic variations
  - Utilization of immunological proteins to gain entry into host cells, e.g. utilization of complement proteins by *Trypanosoma* and
  - Development—stage specific antigen expression to evade immune processing, e.g. malarial parasite.
- Various parasites elicit generation of different types of immune response but typically the levels of immunoglobulins in the serum are raised. IgM levels elevate in *Trypanosoma* infection and malaria; IgG in malaria and visceral leichmaniasis and IgE in worm infections.
- In general terms, cell-mediated immune response is are more effective against the intracellular protozoa, whereas antibody is more effective against extracellular parasites in blood and tissue fluids.
- Antibody alone or with complement can damage some extracellular parasites, but it is more effective in combination with certain effector cells like macrophages (which gets activated by complement proteins and mediates opsonization) or natural killer cells which promote antibody dependent cell cytotoxicity.
- Within a single infection of parasite, different immune responses may act against different development stages of the parasite. In malaria, while antibody against the extracellular forms block their capacity to invade new cells, cell-mediated immunity prevents the development of the liver stage within hepatocytes.

Role of Effector Cells in Parasitic Infection

- Various types of host effector cells such as macrophages, neutrophils, eosinophils and platelets, help defend the host against parasites and act to control the multiplication and spread of parasites.

- T-cells are fundamental to the control of parasite multiplication. In most parasitic infections, protection can be conferred experimentally on normal animals by the transfer of T-cells from immune animals. The type of T-cell responsible for controlling infection varies according to the parasite nature and stage of infection. For example *Leishmania* infection is countered by CD4 T-cells whereas malarial infection needs both CD4 and CD8 T-cells.
- Many of the anti-parasitic activities of these effector cells are enhanced by cytokines produced in response to the infection, which are essentially produced by T-cells and macrophages.
- Macrophages not only act as APC to the parasitic antigens, they also affect the course of parasitic infections in two ways:
  1. They act as effector cells which inhibit the multiplication of parasites and destroy them and
  2. They secrete molecules such as IL-1, TNF-α, TGF-β and prostaglandins which regulate the inflammatory response.
- Phagocytosis by macrophages is important against smaller parasites and its effectiveness is markedly enhanced by opsonization of the parasite by the antibodies and the complement C3b, leading to more rapid clearance of the protozoan parasites from the blood.
- Other granulocytes like neutrophils and eosinophils also contribute to protection against parasites. Neutrophils kill parasites by both oxygen-dependent and oxygen-independent pathways, including NO-mediated cell death. Neutrophils are present in the parasite infected lesions and are involved in the clearing of parasites from the bursting cells.
- Eosinophilia and production of high levels of IgE are typical hallmarks of infection by parasitic worms. IgE-dependent mast cell reaction has evolved primarily to localize the eosinophils near the parasite and enhance their anti-parasitic action.
- Mast cells have preformed mediators in their cytoplasm, which are released upon activation from antigen-activated T-cells in worm infections.
- Platelets are capable of killing various types of parasites including the schistosoma stage of flukes. Their cytotoxic activities are enhanced by cytokines.

Chapter 7

Inflammation and Hypersensitivities

HYPERSENSITIVITY

- An inappropriate or exaggerated adaptive immune response is termed hypersensitivity. Inflammation and tissue damage may occur. Depending upon mediators and mechanisms there can be four types of hypersensitivity.

Table 7.1: Types of hypersensitivities and their immunological mechanism

Feature	*Hypersensitivity type*			
	Type I	*Type II*	*Type III*	*Type IV*
Immune reactant	IgE	IgG	IgG	T_H1/ T_H2/ CTL
Antigen/ allergen	Soluble antigen	Soluble antigen	Soluble antigen	Soluble antigen or cell associated antigen
Effector mechanism	Mast cell activation	Activation of phagocytes and NK cells	Complement mediated damage and neutrophils	Macrophage and eosinophil activation and cell cytotoxicity
Examples	Allergic rhinitis, asthma	Drug allergies	Serum sickness, arthus reaction	Contact dermatitis, tuberculin reaction

I. Type I Hypersensitivity (Anaphylaxis or Immediate Hypersensitivity)

- 'Allergy', a term coined by von Pirquet in 1906, means a hypersensitive response by genetically susceptible individuals to small amounts of antigen (allergen) to which they have already been sensitized. Common allergens are pollens, moulds, insect venom, dust foreign serum and penicillin.
- Initial exposure to allergen by inhalation, ingestion, injection or insect sting leads to excess IgE production and its binding to the Fc receptor on the surface of mast cells and basophils. IgE antibody does not cross the placenta although there is a hereditary disposition to sensitization. $F(ab')_2$ of these antibodies on mast cell surface remain free to bind allergen.
- A local response is termed '**Atopy**' (e.g. urticaria, asthma and allergic rhinitis) and a systemic response '**Anaphylaxis**'.

Mechanism of Type I Hypersensitivity

- On re-exposure of sensitized host to the allergen, binding to cell-linked IgE antibodies occurs.
- This aggregates several such antibodies and this membrane perturbation causes degranulation of the mast cells.
- Release of pharmacologically reactive substances like histamine, leukotrienes, serotonin and bradykinin, etc. from the mast cell granules have varied effects on various tissues
  a. *Effect on GI tract*: Increased fluid secretion and peristalisis leading to expulsion of GI tract contents (diarrhea or vomiting)
  b. *Effect on airways*: Decreased diameter and increased mucus secretion which lead to congestion and blockage of airways (wheezing and cough generation)
  c. *Effect on blood vessels:* Increased blood flow and permeability which cause increased fluid in the tissues causing increased lymph flow to lymph nodes and increased presence cells and proteins in the tissues leading to edema.

Properties of Type I Allergen

- The typical characteristics of allergen which are taken by inhalation route should include:

Table 7.2: Molecules released by mast cells on activation and their biological effects

Class of the molecule	*Example*	*Effect*
Enzyme	Tryptase; cathepsin G, chymase	Remodelling of connective tissue matrix
Toxic mediator	Histamine; heparin	Toxic to parasites Increase in vascular permeability Smooth muscle contraction
Cytokines	IL-4; IL-13	Stimulation and amplification of T_H2 response
	IL-3, IL-5; GM-CSF	Eosinophil production and activation
	TNF-α	Promotes inflammation; cytokine production and activation of endothelium
Chemokine	MIP-1α	Attracts monocytes, macrophages and neutrophils to the site of activation
Lipid mediators	Leukotrienes C4, D4 and E4	Smooth muscle contraction Increases vascular permeability Stimulation of mucus secretion
	Platelet-activating factor	Attracts leukocytes Amplification in production of lipid mediators Activation of neutrophils, eosinophils and platelets

a. *Protein* only acts as allergens by this route
b. The proteins have to be *enzymatically active* and should preferably a protease
c. The allergen is encountered in *low dose* which favors activation of IL-4 producing T-cells.
d. It generally has *low molecular weight* so it can diffuse into the mucus from the allergen particle.
e. It has *solubility* so it is rapidly released from the particle
f. It is generally *very stable* so it survives in the dessicated particle and

g. It contains *peptides that bind to the host MHC II* so it can prime the host T-cells.

Examples of Type I Hypersensitivity

- Urticaria (hives) is a cutaneous form of type I hypersensitivity and is characterized by a wheal and flare lesion due to histamine release. This leads to vasodilation and increased vascular permeability of the skin.

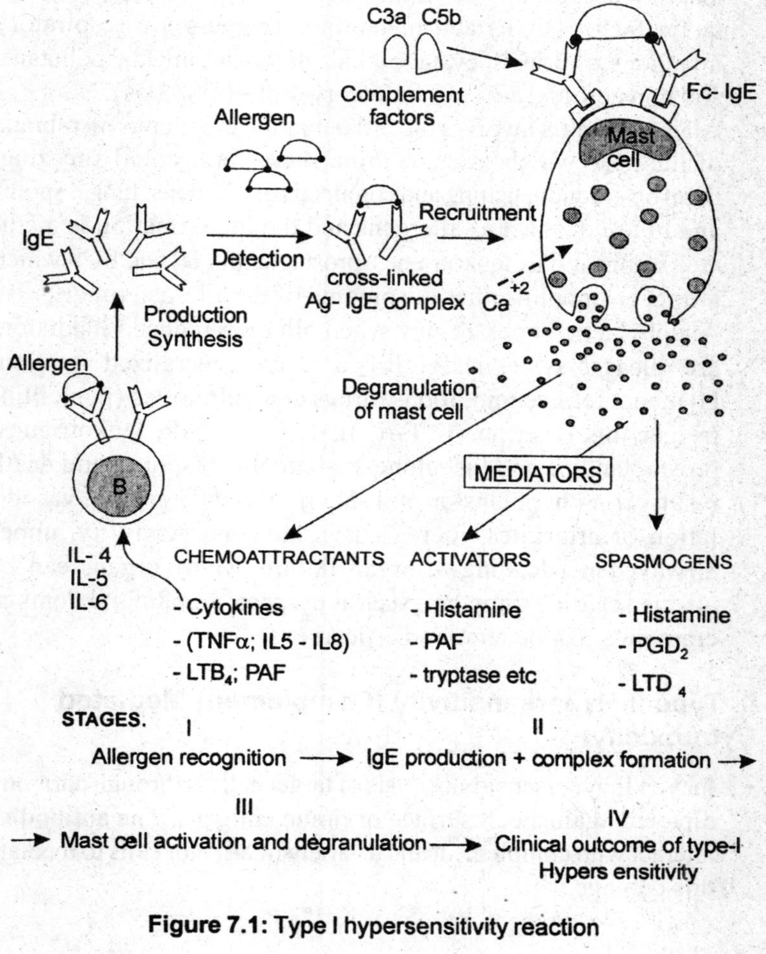

Figure 7.1: Type I hypersensitivity reaction

- Asthma is characterized by airway obstruction resulting in acute respiratory distress including wheezing, dyspnea, chest tightness and cough. Extrinsic asthma is caused by chronic exposure to occupational, environmental and food allergens whereas intrinsic asthma can be induced by nonimmunologic means. Influx of mast cells, $CD4^+$ cells, T_H2 cells, basophils and eosinophils leads to inflammation. Following the allergen—IgE union, mucus secretion and mediator induced obstruction of the smooth muscle surrounding the vacuoles cause obstruction. Mediators are the leukotrienes, platelet-activating factor (PAF), eosinophil chemotactic factor (ECF) and histamine. Triggers are respiratory infections, aspirin, isocyanate inhalants, environmental pollutants and nonsteroidal anti-inflammatory drugs (NSAIDs).
- Allergic rhinitis involves the inflammation of mucous membrane of the nose which leads to rhinorrhea, paroxysmal sneezing, nasal obstruction, itching and conjunctivitis. Pollens, fungal spores and house dust act as allergens and the inflammation is mediated by histamine, leukotrienes, prostaglandin D_2 and ECF which attract eosinophils after the binding of the allergen to IgE.
- Anaphylactic shock occurs when allergen-induced mediators are released systemically. It is a severe generalized reaction. Hymenoptera venom, foods, drugs and antibiotics (penicillin) trigger this reaction. TNF-α, IL-1, IL-6, PAF, leukotrienes, prostaglandins and histamine mediate this response and death results from hypotension and shock caused by general vasodilation of arterioles, increased vascular permeability, upper airwayedema leading to organ failure. Many organs can be affected causing symptoms such as dyspnea, vomiting, abdominal cramping, angioedema and urticaria.

II. Type II Hypersensitivity (Complement Mediated Cytotoxicity)

- In type II hypersensitivity, lysis of target cells is through antibody directed against cell surface or tissue antigens. The antibodies interact with complement and a variety of effector cells to mediate this damage.

- Target cells may be blood cells and platelets as in transfusion reactions, hemolytic disease of the newborn, autoimmune hemolytic anemia and drug induced hypersensitivity or tissue antigens as in Goodpasture's syndrome and myasthenia gravis.
- Reactions to cellular antigens and hyperacute graft rejections are also examples of this type of hypersensitivity.

Mechanism of Type II Hypersensitivity

- Target cells are linked to effector cells, such as macrophages, neutrophils, eosinophils and K-cells by means of Fc receptors on these effector cells.
- Activation of C1 of the classical complement pathway on interaction with antibodies bound to target cells can lead to lysis through the deposition of the C5b-9 membrane attack complex on the target cells.
- Complement protein C3b and its fragment C3d, bound to target cells during the classical pathway of activation, can act as recognition structures for effector cells carrying complement receptors.
- Opsonization of the target cell or microorganism with the help of IgG and complement fragments helps phagocytic action of effector cells.
- Lysosomal activity of the phagocytes and their capacity to produce reactive oxygen species is also increased in this process.
- Complement fragment C5a, fibrin peptides, leukotrienes and chemotactic peptides from mast cells and lymphocytes help in attracting phagocytes to the site of hypersensitivity reaction.
- Binding of antibody to Fc receptor on the phagocyte stimulates them to release arachidonic acid, precursor for production of prostaglandins and leukotrienes involved in inflammation. K-cells bind antibody through their high affinity Fc receptor and act like cytotoxic T-cells.

Examples of Type II Hypersensitivity

- *Transfusion reactions* arise after the transfusion of blood containing RBC antigens foreign to the recipient. ABO incompatibility occurs between antigen and preformed antibodies

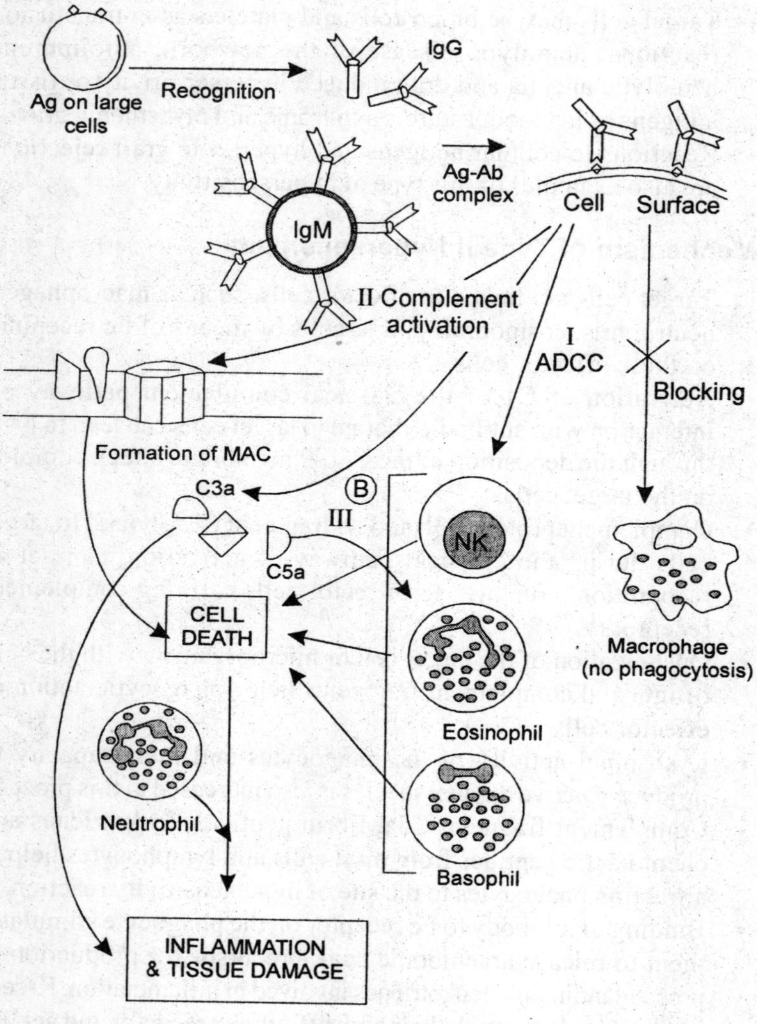

Figure 7.2: Type II hypersensitivity reaction

in the recipient's blood causing the donor's RBCs to agglutinate. Rapid phagocytosis or complement mediated RBC lysis follow.

- *Hemolytic disease of the newborn* (erythroblastosis fetalis) is caused by the placental transfer of the maternal anti-Rh IgG antibody which binds to Rh^+ fetal erythrocytes leading to rapid phagocytosis or complement mediated RBC lysis. Hemolysis causes hemoglobinuria and conversion to indirect bilirubin. Accumulation of indirect bilirubin leads to respiratory and brain damage.

- *Goodpasture's syndrome* is characterized by glomerulonephritis and pulmonary hemorrhage. The antigen is a glycoprotein spread uniformly on the glomerular basement membrane (GBM). Hosts produce IgG antibody which binds to the membrane antigen and activates complement, releasing chemotactic factor C5a. This attracts the neutrophils to the antibody-GBM complex, where they release lysosomal enzymes. These enzymes cause severe necrosis of the glomeruli and a loss of filtration capacity.

III. Type III Hypersensitivity (Antigen- Antibody Complex Mediated Hypersensitivity)

- Deposition of Ag-Ab complexes of small size, circulating after escaping phagocytosis, on tissue or on the surface of blood vessels leads to type III hypersensitivity.
- Multiple forms of this response exist, depending upon the type and location of antigen and how it interacts with the antibody. However, the outcome always depends on complement and granulocytes which bring about tissue injury. If the site is a glomerular basement membrane, loss of integrity and release of proteins and red cells into urine results; and if the site is a joint meniscus, destruction of synovial membranes and cartilage occurs.
- The antibodies may be against antigens like DNA, insulin, thyroglobulin, group A nephritogenic streptococci and foreign serum.

Mechanism of Type III Hypersensitivity

- *Stage 1.* The deposited Ag-Ab complexes activate complement and release chemotactic factors C3a and C5a, anaphylotoxins and clotting factors causing a local increase in vessel permeability and permits the release of serum (edema).

- *Stage 2.* Neutrophils are attracted to the area of deposition and release lysosomal enzymes that attack the tissue and cause hemorrhage and necrosis.

Table 7.3: Types of immune complex diseases

Cause	*Antigen*	*Site of complex deposition*
Persistent infection	Microbial antigens	Infected organ(s), kidney
Autoimmunity	Self - antigens	Kidney, joint, arteries, skin
Inhaled antigen	Mould, plant or animal antigens	Lung

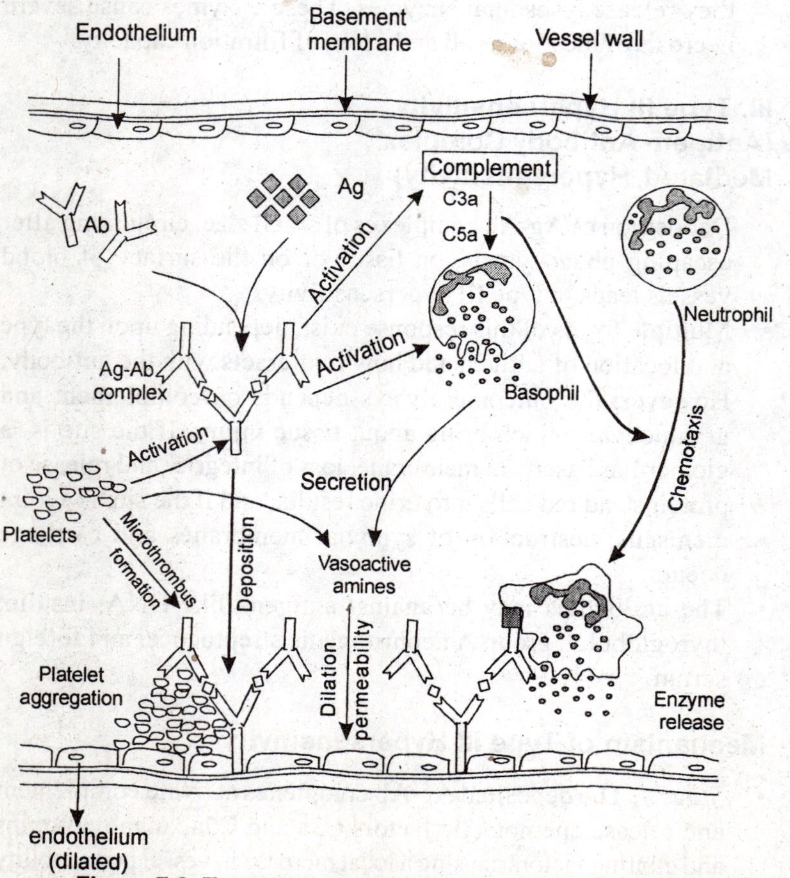

Figure 7.3: Type III hypersensitivity reaction in a capillary

Examples of Ag-Ab Complex Reactions

- *Arthus reaction* is a rare, severe inflammatory response to gross intravascular Ag-Ab precipitates of intermediate size. Complement-mediated chemotactic factors C3a, C5a, polymorphoneuclear neutrophil (PMN) infiltration, and platelets result in hemorrhagic, necrotic lesions..
- *Serum sickness* is a complement-dependent systemic immune complex reaction caused by injection of foreign serum or its products. A milder allergic vasculitis can be elicited by drugs like sulphonamides, cephalosporins or thiourea. Symptoms of serum sickness include fever, rash, lymphadenopathy and joint pain.
- *Polyarteritis nodosa* is characterized by the effect on arterial walls by the deposition of circulating Ag-Ab complexes, causing thrombosis and obliteration of blood flow. Frequently, hepatitis-B antibody complexes are involved.
- *Glomerulonephritis* is an inflammatory response caused by deposition of soluble Ag-Ab complexes which deposit on and behind the renal GBM. Loss of filtration capacity and destruction of the glomeruli is achieved through release of enzymes by neutrophils attracted to the GBM.
- *Systemic lupus erythematosus* (SLE) is characterized by the formation of autoantibodies to many endogenous antigens like, RBCs, WBCs, platelets, double stranded RNA (dsRNA) and anti-dsDNA. It is a chronic inflammatory disease usually affecting young women between 20-45 years of age. It may be initiated by an antibody response against bacterial or viral DNA, followed by loss of regulatory control of self-tolerance. Symptoms of SLE include polyarthralgia or arthritis. An UV light induced skin rash, facial 'butterfly rash' pleurisy, pericarditis or vasculitis may also be present.
- *Rheumatoid arthritis* is a recurrent inflammatory disease occurring due to local antibody formation in the synovium against an unknown antigen. HLA-DR4 haplotype seems to be more susceptible to this disease. Ag-Ab interaction alters the tertiary structure of the antibody, revealing previously buried amino-acid sequences 'foreign' to the immune system. These new

epitopes stimulate the local production of an antibody (usually IgM), called rheumatoid factor. The antibody can react with the Fc domain of the IgG molecules (antibody against an antibody). IgM-IgG complexes form in the synovial fluid and activate complement and chemokines. Lysosomal enzymes released by the neutrophils destroy articular cartilage. Macrophages release IL-1, IL-6 and TNF-α and osteoclasts, which injure bone. Inflammation of the pannus and loss of cartilage cause joint lesions. Rheumatoid factor can be detected by latex agglutination tests, where IgG-coated latex particles are added to the patient's serum.

IV. Type IV Hypersensitivity (Delayed Type Hypersensitivity-DTH)

- Type IV or delayed type hypersensitivity is the consequence of cell-mediated immunity and is typically used as a general category to describe all those hypersensitivity reactions which take more than 12 hours to develop and which do not involve humoral immune response.
- The responses can be passively transferred with an appropriate quantity of T-cells and cannot be transferred from one animal to another through serum.
- Essentially, three types of type IV hypersensitivity reactions are recognized on the basis of reaction they produce when antigen was applied directly to the skin or injected intradermally. The degree and reactivity is assessed by measuring the thickening of the skin.
  a. Contact hypersensitivity-takes 48–72 hours to develop
  b. Tuberculin–type hypersensitivity–also takes 48-72 hours to develop and
  c. Granulamatous reactions which develops after 21-28 days.

Mechanism of Type IV Hypersensitivity

- Tissue damage results from excess activation of macrophages by cytokines from $CD4^+$, T_H1, and $CD8^+$ cells.
- CMI is initiated by the reaction of T-cells with the antigen that is presented in association with MHC class II molecules on APCs.

- This leads to proliferation of the T-cells and the release of several lymphokines, causing non-specific accumulation and activation of monocytes and macrophages.
- Macrophages ingest and cause destruction by released enzymes or by direct attack on invading cells.
- In addition to tuberculin-type reactions, contact sensitivity, allograft rejection and the GVH response are examples where CMI is involved in type IV hypersensitivity.

Example of Type IV Hypersensitivity

- *Contact hypersensitivity*, it is characterized clinically by an eczematous reaction at the site of contact with the allergen. In most of these cases, the allergen is typically a hapten which itself cannot mount an effective immune response but can penetrate the epidermis wherein covalently conjugates with the normal body proteins. The Langerhan's cells, derived from follicular dendritic cells, are the primary APC in contact hypersensitivity. They are located in the superbasal epidermis and express typical cell surface markers of APC such as CD1m MHC II antigens and surface receptors for Fc and complement. The hapten-protein complex is taken up by these cells and is processed and presented to $CD4^+$ T cells. This leads to activation of T-cell which stimulates kertinocytes leading to consequential secretion of proinflammatory cytokines such as IL-1, IL-6 and GM-CSF.
- *Tuberculin-type hypersensitivity* was originally described by Koch. It was generated when a purified lipoprotein antigen derived from tubercle bacilli was injected subcutaneously under the skin of tuberculosis patients. The reaction essentially generated fever and generalized sickness, followed by development of an area of generalized thickness, redness and swelling at the site of injection. Such reaction was also generated using purified protein derivatives of other bacteria such as *M. leprae* and *Leishmania tropica* in sensitized individuals. Such type of hypersensitivity may also be induced by certain nonmicrobial antigens such as beryllium and zirconium.
- *Granulamatous hypersensitivity* is clinically the most important form delayed hypersensitivity. It usually results from persistence

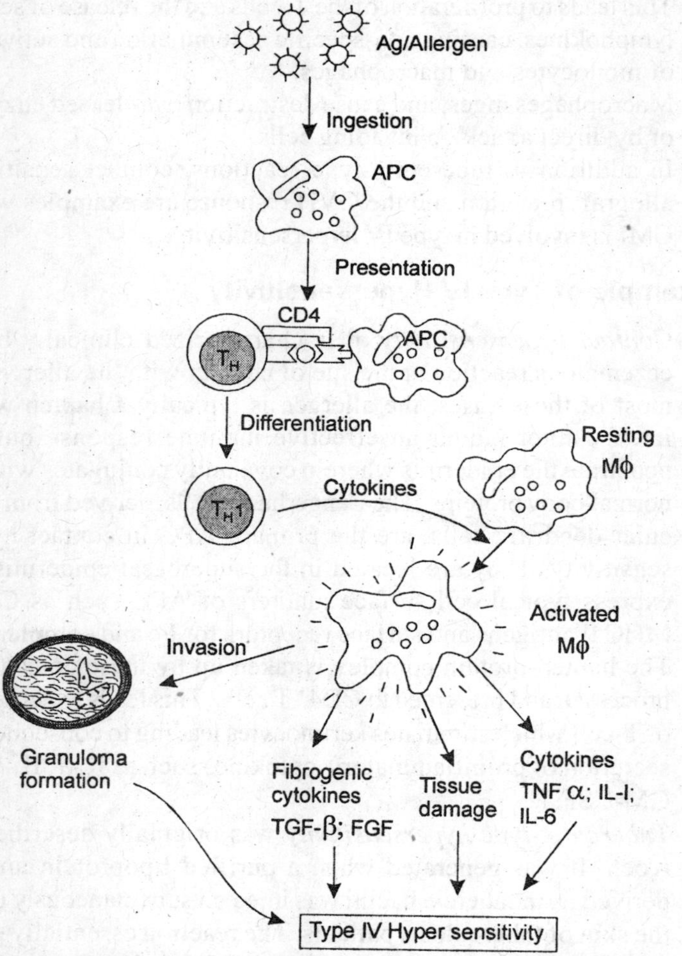

Figure 7.4: Generation of type-IV or delayed type of hypersensitivity through T_H1-cells

of microorganism or other particles within macrophages which the cell is unable to destroy. The reaction typically involve formation of localized encapsulated 'granuloma' containing these cells infected with persistent antigens. Many diseases manifest the onset of delayed type hypersensitivity such as tuberculosis, leprosy, leishmaniasis, listeriosis, deep fungal infections and helminthic diseases such as schistosomiasis.

Chapter 8

Autoimmune and Immunodeficiency Disorders

I. AUTOIMMUNE DISORDERS

- A cell–mediated or antibody-mediated *immune response against the self* is termed as an autoimmune disorder.
- In a normal individual, the anti-self response is suppressed by various mechanism
  a. *Clonal deletion:* During the B-cell or T-cell development, the self-reactive cells undergo deletion in bone marrow or thymus respectively. This process takes place through specific and selective apoptosis of these cells when they encounter self–antigens during their development.
  b. *Clonal anergy:* This phenomenon describes the loss of functions of T- and B-cells if antigens are presented to them without MHC or without the costimulatory signals.
  c. *Tolerance*: It is immunological unresponsiveness to self-antigens. The B-cells against such self-antigens do exist in the clonal lineage.
  d. *Peripheral suppression:* It is elicited if tolerogenic amounts of an antigen is administered or when $CD8^+$ T-cells or macrophages secrete the down regulatory cytokines such as TGF-β.

Breakdown of any of these processes can lead to development of autoimmune disorder.

Development of Autoimmune Disorders

- Breakdown of these processes can take place through many mechanisms which include:
  a. *Cross-reaction of microbial antigens with self-antigens*. Hence, after the initial exposure to the exogenous antigen, the immune system mounts response to the similar self-antigens. For example Staphylococcal antigens cross-react with sarcolemmel heart muscles and kidney; anti-DNA antibodies developed against the pathogen DNA and turn against self-DNA as well (as in SLE-systemic lupus erythematosus).
  b. *Development of new antigenic determinants*-Followed by the processes such as clonal selection and maturity, many antigenic proteins undergo variations and development much later in life and hence they might not be eliminated from the immune-cell's clonal pool during development. For example, rheumatoid arthritis is essential development of antibodies against Fc region of IgG antibodies, the antigenicity of whose changes after combination with antigens in synovial complex.

Types of Autoimmune Disorders

- Depending the organs which are affected by the development of autoantibodies, the autoimmune disorders are classified in *generalized or systemic* disorders or *organ specific* disorder.
- Though clinically this classification is valid but there exists a tremendous amount of overlap amongst these disorders and their causes.
- Systemic disorders include:
  a. *SLE* which clinically leads to development of erythematous rash, vasculitis and arthritis. Caused by multiple autoreactive antibodies (specially against DNA and nuclear matrix).
  b. *Rheumatoid arthritis* characterized by granulated tissue and subcutaneous nodule formation in the joints. Caused by development of antibodies against immunoglobulins.

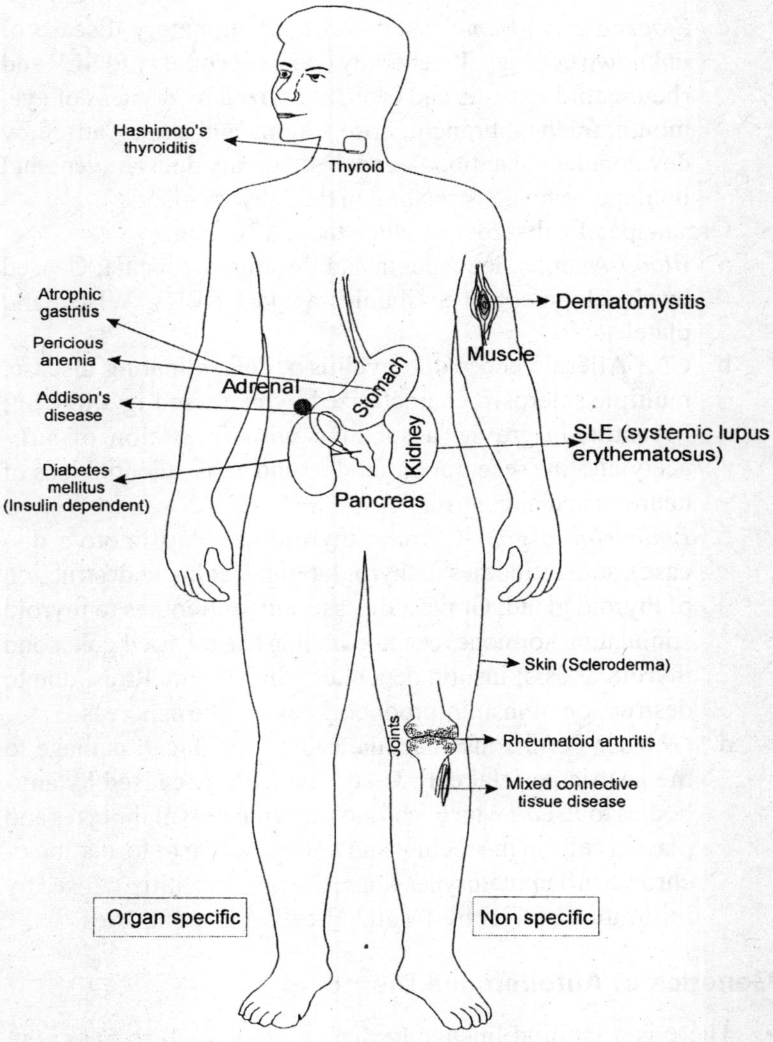

Figure 8.1 Types of autoimmune disorders

Figure 8.1: Types of autoimmune disorders

c. *Sjögren's syndrome* is a chronic inflammatory disease of unknown etiology. It generally occurs secondary to SLE and rheumatoid arthritis and is characterized by dryness of eye, mouth, trachea, bronchi, nose, vagina and skin. Caused by development of antibodies against salivary duct antigens and immune complex formation in the salivary glands.

- Organ-specific disorders include those affecting:

a. *Blood*-Anemia, leucopenia and thrombocytopenia. Caused by development of antibodies against RBCs, WBCs and platelets.

b. *CNS*-Allergic encephalomyelitis, a demyelinating disease; multiple sclerosis, characterized by increased IgG in CSF; Myasthenia gravis, associated with formation of anti-acetylcholine receptor antibodies and consequential loss of neuromuscular control.

c. *Endocrine organs*-Chronic thyroiditis (Hashimoto's disease), autoantibodies to thyroglobulin leading to destruction of thyroid gland; Graves' disease, autoantibodies to thyroid stimulating hormone receptor leading to a diffused goiter and thyrotoxicosis; insulin dependent diabetes mellitus, due to destruction of insulin-producing cells in the pancreas.

d. *GI tract*-Pernicious anaemia, caused by T-cell damage to the gactric parietal cell; Ulcerative colitis, caused by antibodies to *E. coli* which leads to filtration of lymphocytes and plasma cells in the rectum and colon leading to formation of chronic inflammatory leasions; Chronic hepatitis, caused by infiltration of liver by T-cells, B-cells and monocytes.

Genetics of Autoimmune Disorders

- There is a familial linkage to the autoimmune disorders with essentially organ-specific disorders showing hereditary lineage.
- This is perhaps due to association of disorder causing haplotypes to certain restricted MHC classes which is genetically linked.
- A number of autoimmune disorders can be transferred across placenta by pathogenic IgG antibodies. These diseases are caused mostly by autoantibodies to cell surface or tissue matrix

molecules. Such diseases include myasthenia gravis, Graves' disease, thrombocytopenic purpura, neonatal lupus rash or congenital heart block and pemphigus vulgaris.

Treatment of Autoimmune Disorders

- Often for organ-specific disorders, the symptoms can be corrected by metabolic control. For example hypothyroidism can be corrected by administering thyroxine; pernicious anemia by vitamin B_{12} and in others as well.
- In systemic disorders, immunosuppressive therapy along with anti-mitotic drugs can be used to dampen the reaction (not recommended as may cause multiple infections).

II. IMMUNODEFICIENCY DISORDERS

- Immunodeficiencies occur when one or more components of the immune system is defective.
- Most of the immunodeficiency disorders are inherited (*inherited immunodeficiency*) in nature and are usually seen in clinic as cases with recurrent and overwhelming infections.
- The *acquired immunodeficiency* disorders are less common and can be because of malnutrition besides from infections for certain pathogens. Although the pathogenesis of many of these acquired disorders have remained fuzzy, some are caused by known agents, such as drugs or irradiations which damage lymphocytes or by infection with measles or HIV, the causative organism of AIDS.

Types of Immunodeficiency Disorders

a. *Inherited immunodeficiency* diseases are caused by recessive gene defects and for this reason many of the known immunodeficiencies are caused by mutations on the genes on X-chromosome. Since, recessive defects cause disease only when both chromosomes are defective. However, males have only one X-chromosome, hence all males which inherit a X- chromosome carrying the defective gene manifests the disease.

Table 8.1: List of various inherited human immunodeficiency diseases, their causes and their outcome on disease susceptibility.

Deficiency Disorder	*Specific genetic abnormality/ies*	*Susceptibility*
SCID (Severe combined immunodeficiency disorder)	ADA deficiency PNP deficiency X-linked scid deficiency Autosomal *scid* DNA repair defect	General
DiGeorge's syndrome	Thymic aplasia	General
MHC class I immuno-deficiency	Mutation associated with TAP (transporters associated with antigen processing)	Chronic lung and skin infection
MHC class II immuno-deficiency	Lack of expression of MHC II	General
Wiskott-Aldrich syndrome	X-linked, defective WASP gene	To encapsulated extra-cellular bacteria
X-linked agammaglo-bulinemia	Loss of *blk* tyrosine kinase	To extracellular bacteria and viruses
X-linked hyper-IgM syndrome	Defective CD40 ligand	Extracellular bacteria
Common variable immunodeficiency	Unknown; MHC-linked	Extracellular bacteria
Selective IgA	Unknown; MHC-linked	Respiratory infections
Phagocyte deficiencies	Many different	Extracellular bacteria and fungi
Complement deficiencies	Many different	Extracellular bacteria specially *Neisseria* spp.
Natural killer cell defect	Unknown	Herpes virus
X-linked lymphopro-liferative syndrome	SH2D1A mutation	B-cell tumors driven or mediated by EBV
Bloom's syndrome	Defect in DNA helicase	Respiratory infections

b. *Acquired immunodeficiency syndrome* (AIDS) is characterized by a susceptibility to infection with oppurtunistic pathogens, development of aggressive form of Kaposi's sarcoma or B-cell lymphoma, accompanied with a severe reduction in the count of CD4 T-cells.

- The disease is caused by an RNA reterovirus, human immunodeficiency virus (HIV) which selectively infects the $CD4^+$ T cells (T helper cells) of the immune system.
- Most individuals infected with HIV progress over time to AIDS.
- The primary infection with HIV is asymptomatic in ½ of the cases. In other half of the cases, an influenza-like illness with abundance of virus in the peripheral blood and a marked reduction in the number of CD4 T-cells takes place.
- This acute viremia is associated with recruitment of $CD8^+$ Tc cells, which kill the HIV infected cells and bring about the reduction in the virus levels in the blood.
- The reduction in viral levels in the blood is not a hallmark of 'curing' of HIV rather it leads to a stage of clinical quiescence also known clinically as latency or the asymptomatic period. This period is not silent, however, as there is a persistent replication of the virus which leads to a gradual decline in the counts and function of $CD4^+$ T-cells. Once the minimal threshold count of T cells is achieved, which might take anything from 2-15 years from primary infection, the people infected with HIV ends up developing AIDS.
- Although viral load and turnover are usually measured by detecting the viral RNA present in the viral particles in the blood, the major reservoir of the HIV infection is in lymphoid tissue, in which infected $CD4^+$ T-cells, monocytes, macrophages and dendritic cells are found.
- Although most people infected with HIV go on to develop AIDS and ultimately die because of opportunistic infections or cancer, a small percentage of people seroconvert leading to development of antibodies against HIV proteins and are ultimately able to prevent development of progressive disease. That actual process which helps them in becoming seropositive in under intense scrutiny and might provide a lead for developing an effective vaccine against HIV in future.
- Drugs which block the replication of HIV (for it being a RNA virus it needs a reverse transcriptase, which can form the target of drugs) leading to rapid decerase in the titer of infectious virus and an increase in $CD4^+$ cell count.

- HIV accumulates many mutations in the course of infection in an individual and drug treatment might follow with outgrowth of drug-resistant variants of the virus. This is very critical as HIV has a very high replication rate (approximately 10^9 to 10^{10} virions are generated everyday) along with a very high mutation frequency (~ 3×10^{-5} mutations per nucleotide per replication cycle), a high number of variants can be developed in a single day which might interfere with the therapy outcome.

Table 8.2: A list of categories and examples of opportunistic pathogens which kills AIDS patients.

Category of opportunistic disorder	*Examples*
Extracellular infection	Parasitic infection
	Toxoplasma spp.
	Cryptosporidium spp.
	Leishmania spp.
	Microsporidium spp.
Intracellular bacteria infection	*Mycobacterium tuberculosis*
	M. intracellulare
	M. avium
	Salmonella spp.
Fungal infections	*Pneumocystis carinii*
	Cryptococcus neoformans
	Candida spp.
	Histoplama capsulatum
Viral infections	Herpes simplex
	Cytomegalovirus
	Varicella zoster
Malignancies	Kaposi's sarcoma
	Non-Hodgkin's lymphoma
	Burkitt's lymphoma
	Primary lymphoma of the brain

Chapter 9

Applications of Immunology in Medicine

I. TRANSPLANTATION IMMUNOLOGY

Transplantation biology as a discipline of medicine rests entirely on two singular aspects '*acceptance or rejection*' of the graft.

- The acceptance or the rejection of the graft is determined by the compatibility between the histocompatibility antigens (also termed as human leukocyte antigens or HLAs) of the host and donor.
- HLA have two major functions:
  a. Major physiological function is to bind and present processed foreign antigenic molecules to the T-cells, thus triggering an immune response (as MHC).
  b. They also provide discrimination or distinction capabilities of immune cells to distinguish self from non-self cells or antigens. *Any cells expressing a different set of MHC (by virtue of it being a transplanted organ/ cell, it would be expressing the HLA antigens of the donor) would be essentially treated as a foreign cell only and an appropriate immune response would be mounted against it, which would ultimately decide the graft acceptance (milder or no response) or rejection (strong response).*

- HLAs are classified in two distinct categories essentially on the basis of their presence on various cell types and their antigen presentation properties.
  a. *Class I antigens* (MHC - I) are present on all nucleated cells and have three gene loci termed as HLA-A,B and C. They can be serologically defined using anti-HLA antibodies. They present the processed antigens to Tc ($CD8^+$) cells and present peptides of 8–10 amino acids.
  b. *Class II antigens* (MHC-II) are present on immune effector cells (essentially all antigen presenting cells; B-cells, macrophages; etc). Similar to HLA class I antigens they also have three gene loci, all within HLA-D region termed as HLA-DP, DQ and DR. They present foreign antigens to T_H ($CD4^+$) cells.
- The MHC molecules have distinct subunit constitution and structures
  a. MHC I molecule is a heterodimer of a membrane spanning α-chain of 43 kDa bound non-covalently to β_2-microglobulin protein of 12 kDa which does not span the membrane. The α-chain folds into three distinct domains α_1, α_2 and α_3. The α_3 domain and β_2 microglobulin proteins show similarity to the immunoglobulin fold and have similar structures. The folding of α_1 and α_2 domain form the long cleft or groove wherein the peptide or antigen binds.
  b. The MHC-II protein consists of two transmembrane glycoprotein chains α-chain of 34 kDa and β-chain of 29 kDa. Each chain has two domain and all the four domains form the compact four domain structure typical of MHC-I. Similar to the MHC-I, the α_2 and β_2 domains have structural characteristics similar to that of immunoglobulins and form the characteristic immunoglobulin fold. The peptide binding cleft is created by all the domains and is characteristically open at both ends.

Histocompatibility Analysis in Transplantation

- It is of importance to analyze and match the donor and recipient HLA antigens to improve the graft acceptability. On the basis

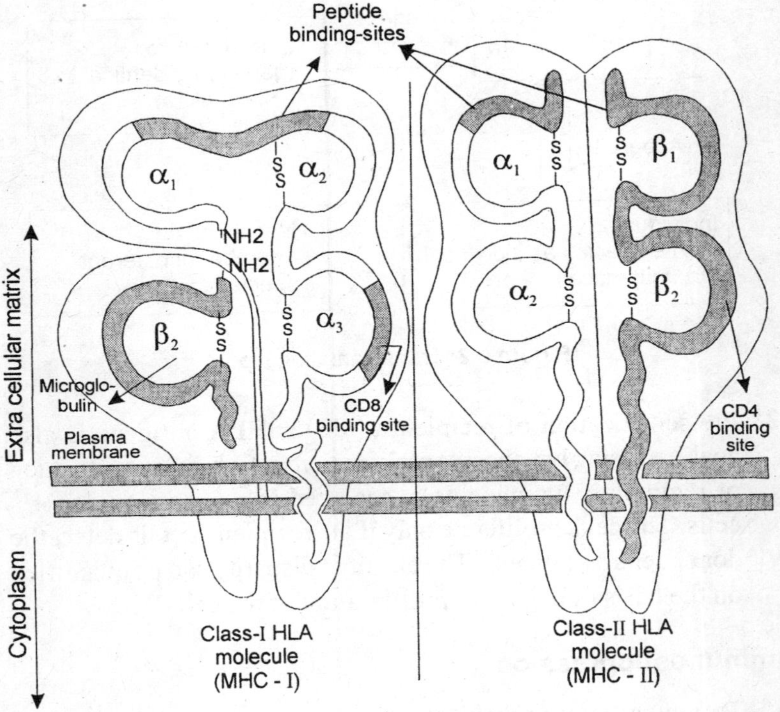

Figure 9.1: Structure of class I and class II human leukocyte antigen (HLA) molecules

of the similarity between the HLA antigens between the donor and the recipients, the grafts are classified as *autograft* (same HLA), *isograft* (HLA matching), allograft (HLA similar) and xenograft (no match). Amongst all the grafts the autograft and isografts are mostly accepted and others are rejected by the recipient.

Tests for Typing for HLA Compatibility

1. HLA gene loci can be sequenced and their profiles can be matched. Alternatively the HLA-typing can be performed using the anti-HLA serum (Specific against various serotypes).
2. The blood group antigens, *viz.* ABO and Rh-factors are also analyzed.

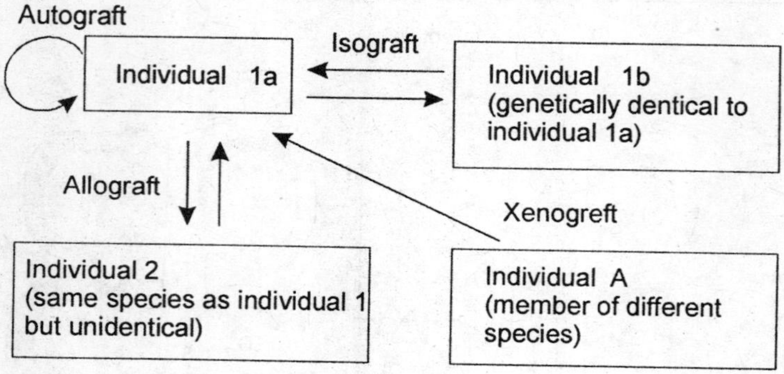

Figure 9.2: Transplantation types

3. Pre-sensitization of recipient to donor HLA antigens is also analyzed using lymphocyte proliferation test wherein proliferation of recipient's lymphocyte is analyzed in response to donor's cells. The cells proliferate only if the recipient's cells detect the donor cells as antigens. The extent of disparity can be quantified on the basis of degree of proliferation of the cells.

Immunosuppression

- To increase the probability of graft acceptance the recipients are generally subjected to drugs which act as immune suppressants. Such drugs include:
  a. *Cyclosporin A*–It acts by blocking the synthesis of IL-2 mRNA hence leading to shutdown of the critical T-cell response.
  b. *Rapamycin*–It captures the proliferating T-cells in the G1-phase by binding to essential cyclophilins. It is provided in conjunction with cyclosporine as it does not have any effect on preactivated cells which are inactivated by rapamycin.
  c. *FK 506 (Tacrolimus)*–A macrolide compound which also blocks the IL-2 mRNA synthesis.
  d. *Mycophenolate mofetil* inhibits GMP synthesis required by B and T-cells. It inhibits the enzyme monophosphate dehydrogenase which is involved in the synthesis of GMP.

e. *Corticosteroids* are anti-inflammatory agents which work synergistically with cyclosporine A. They also suppress IL-2 synthesis by blocking the release of IL-1 from macrophages.

f. Specific immunosuppressants.
   i. Immunological suppressants-Antibodies against CD3, CD4, CD25, CD5 antigens, etc. would selectively and specifically inhibit the immune reaction from cells expressing these markers (essentially T-cells).
   ii. Coupled toxins-IL-2 coupled to toxins like diptheria toxin can be used to selectively block the IL-2 receptor expressing cells (T-cells) leading to their suppression.

- Due to such a non-specific immunosuppression, the recipient becomes predisposed to infection from various organisms such as *Candida*, *Aspergillus*, and Epstein-Barr virus amongst others. Hence a typical transplantation recipient is kept under strictly sterile conditions to prevent such commensal infections.
- A variety of organs are transplanted routinely in clinical medicine. Three major advances have made it possible to have routine transplantations
  1. The technical skills required for successful organs transplants have been mastered,
  2. Network of transplantation centers have been organized to ensure that the few healthy organs that are available are HLA-typed and matched with suitable recipient as soon as possible and
  3. The use of many strong immunosuppressive drugs like FK506 and cyclosporine A to inhibit the T-cell response have increased the graft survival rates dramatically.
- Amongst the organs which are routinely transplanted in the clinics are kidney, liver, heart, lung, cornea and bone marrow amongst many others.
- Some tissues and organs in the body are immunologically previlege, i.e. tissue grafts placed in these sites often last indefinitely and antigens placed in these sites do not elicit destructive immune response. Such sites include brain, eye, testis, uterus and hamster cheek pouch.

II. ONCOLOGY: ONCOGENES AND IMMUNOTHERAPY

- A malignant tumor growth that spreads locally by invasion and systemically by metastasis is called **cancer**.
- Tumor or cancer immunology deals with the immunologic aspects of the host-tumor relationship and the utilization of immune response for diagnosis, prophylaxis and therapy of tumors.

Oncogenes and TSAs

- Tumors or cancerous cell arise when growth regulating genes (termed as '*proto-oncogenes*') in normal cells undergo mutations because of biological or chemical processes and hence lose their regulatory aspect becoming damaged and consequently causing neoplastic growth. Such altered genes are then termed as '*oncogenes*'.
- *Oncogenes* present in cells cause neoplastic or unregulated growth. p53, ras, c-myc, Bcl-2 and bcr/abl gene fusion are some examples of oncogenes.
- Though cancer is essentially unregulated growth of self-cells, it still leads to development of certain '*tumor-specific antigens*' (TSA). Such antigens arise because of modifications of self-protein due to mutations and hence they are *not exclusive* to the tumor cells and can very well be present on other systemic cells. Such TSA can be present on the tumor cells in either higher amounts or have a different or modified structure. These aspects of TSAs can be effectively utilized for developing therapies against cancers. Examples of such TSA include, alpha-fetoprotein, carcinoembryonic antigen, heat-stable alkaline phosphatase amongst others.

Immune Response to Cancerous Cells and Immunotherapy

A. Immune Response to Cancer

Immune system can recognize the cancerous cells and TSA and hence can mount an *immune response* using different types of cells such as:

1. $CD4^+$ T_H cells-they secrete several cytokines like IL-2 and IFN-γ which lead to activation of cytotoxic T_C cells.
2. $CD8^+$ T_C cells–they are the actual 'mercenaries' of the cancerous cells, they are initiate lysis of cancerous cells through perforin activation.
3. NK cells-they kill cells through ADCC and lyse them post contact. Since they are not MHC restricted and their activity is increased by IFN-γ, IL-2 and IL-12. They are the most potent weapons against the cancerous cells.
4. Macrophages–the central role of macrophages to almost all immune processes is strongly visible here. They 'probably' help in eradication of tumors through their multifaceted armory which includes respiratory burst, NO release, proteinases, TNF-α, and ADCC amongst others.

B. Evasion of Immune Surveillance by Cancer

To *counter* such attacks from the immune system arsenal, the cancerous cells also develop *mechanisms to evade*, they include:

1. Rapid tumor growth which might overwhelm the weaker immune reactions.
2. Since cancerous cells are self-cells, a number of them might be expressing a basal low level of MHC or costimulatory molecules on their surface, hence rendering the T-cell response ineffective.
3. The antibodies which are generated against the TSA could actually be blocking the TSA (if they are not activating the complement) and might be preventing their availability to the T-cells.
4. Many cancerous cells undergo modulation and modification of their TSA (similar to many viruses) and hence can evade the generation of a proper and long lasting immune response.
5. Many tumors/cancers arise in immunologically-restricted site such as eye and CNS, generating a response to such tumors is mostly improbable.
6. Some tumors can be involved in the synthesis of immuno-suppressive molecules such as TGF–β and prostaglandins which block an effective immune response.

C. Immunotherapy Towards Cancer

Development or regression of cancer is the net result of the outcome of the constant tussle between the immune surveillance mechanisms of the host and the counter immune-evading mechanisms of the cancerous cells. To provide support to the immune system in destruction of such cancers many *immunotherapy* modules have been developed over the years.

Immunotherapy essentially implies to the use of cells or modulators of immune system as therapeutic entities to counter an immunological challenge.

A number of immunotherapy setups have been described for cancerous cells, which uses

1. *Lymphokine–activated killer cells* (LAK), tumor reactive cells or unknown lineage. Such cells are isolated from the blood of cancer patient and are reinjected into the bloodstream after *in-vitro* expansion using cytokine IL-2 which elicits its proliferation.
2. *Tumor infiltrating lymphocytes* (TIL), similar to LAK they are also expanded *in-vitro* using IL-2. The difference between TIL and LAK is that TIL are isolated from the tumor bed and consequently can have more specificity than LAKs.
3. *Monoclonal antibodies*, directed against TSA can be utilized to target cancerous cells. Such TSA-specific monoclonal antibodies can be conjugated to prodrugs, toxins, radioisotope, etc. to selectively deliver the therapeutically active entity right into the tumor without having any by-stander toxicity effect of the 'killer' entity.
4. *Cytokines*, to enhance the outcome or the efficacy of CMI response against the cancerous cells.

III. IMMUNIZATION (VACCINATION)

- Immunization is the most effective technique to battle against the infectious disease.
- Immunologically it is generation of an immune system memory to a particular disease using the attenuated or derivatized forms of a disease causing pathogen, which technically cannot cause disease.

Types of Vaccines (Table 9.1)

- The nature and type of vaccine to be used for a disease might differ from the one used for other disease and this is essentially on the basis of the efficacy and success rate of one type of vaccine over the other one. For example, a protein-based vaccine have proved to be largely successful for tetanus but for polio attenuated virions are used.
- Before the use of any new vaccine, the candidate should fulfill some basic criteria for being an effective vaccine. Such criteria include:
  a. *Safety*-The vaccine in itself should not cause disease, illness or death.

Table 9.1: Types of antigenic preparations used as vaccines

Nature of antigen	*Type*	*Example*	*Features*
Living organisms	Live	Vaccinia for small-pox	A single inoculum can provide life-long immunity
	Attenuated	BCG for tuberculosis Polio drops (Salk) MMR (for Mumps, measles and Rubella)	
Intact but non-living organisms	Bacteria	Pertussis; Cholera; Typhoid, etc.	Multiple doses have to be given and needs adjuvant
	Viruses	Polio (Sabin); Rabies; Hepatitis	
Cellular/Sub-cellular fragments of the organisms	Surface antigens Polysaccharides	Hepatitis B Pneumococcus	Repeated vaccination
Toxins		Diptheria; Tetanus	Protection for short-term only
DNA-vaccines	Naked DNA	Experimental stages	Experimental stages but advantages include stability, low
	Expressing DNA	Hepatitis B	cost, ease of production and long – lasting protection

b. *Protection*-It should be able to provide protection from illness resulting from the infection from the live pathogen whenever encountered.
c. *Sustenance*-The protection provided by the vaccine should preferably be long lasting
d. *Neutralizing antibodies production*– Some infections cause destruction of cells which cannot be replaced e.g. polio virus destroys neurons. For such cases it is essential that the vaccine should stimulate production of neutralizing antibodies.
e. T-*cell induction*–Many intracellular pathogens are not cleared by the antibodies and therein the cell-mediated immune response is more suitable. Hence the vaccine should be capable in eliciting a T-cell memory.
f. *Practical considerations*-Should be of low cost, have long shelf life, have ease of administration and have fewer side-effects if any.

Vaccination Schedule

A proper vaccination schedule is now followed for almost all newborn children and a proper administration schedule is now followed in almost all countries, which is listed herein Table 9.2).

Table 9.2: Types of antigenic preparations used as vaccines

Disease	*Vaccine*	*Schdule*
Polio	Salk/ Sabin (Oral Drops)	1st dose-2nd month 2nd dose-4th month 3rd dose-6-18 months Subsequent doses-4-6 years
Hepatitis	Hepatitis B	1st dose-After birth 2nd dose-1st month 3rd dose-6th month
Diptheria-Tetanus-Pertussis	DPT (toxoid)	3 doses between 2-6 months
Mumps Measles Rubella	MMR (attenuated)	12-15 months

- Though a number of diseases are covered in these vaccination schedules, understanding for a number of infectious diseases still have not reached a status wherein an effective vaccine can be developed. This is essentially due to lack of understanding of their immune recognition process using which an effective memory for the disease can be generated.

Such diseases include

- AIDS; caused by *HIV* and have problems associated with antigenic variations and immune suppression mechanisms.
- Tuberculosis caused by *Mycobacterium tuberculosis*. The bacterium resides inside macrophages and hence can effectively evade the immune surveillance mechanisms BCG, the only known vaccine shown variable efficacy hence ineffective.
- Adenovirus and rhinovirus have multiple serotypes hence ineffective as vaccine candidates.
- Malaria, caused by *Plasmodium* have a huge panoply of antigenic repertoire hence have problems associated with antigenic variation.
- Schistosomiasis
- Worm infections
- Diarrheal disease

- **Adjuvants** are substances which are added to vaccines to increase their immunogenicity. Such substances generally preclude rapid release of vaccines (antigens) in the body and consequently 'buys' time for proper recruitment of CMI components namely macrophages and antigen presenting cells. This ultimately leads to generation of a more effective immune response. Such slow release also prevents the toxic effects of the vaccine. Amongst many adjuvants routinely used in animals only aluminium hydroxide gel is approved for human use.

Chapter 10

Practical Immunology

- Utility of immunological tools in the clinic is widespread and finds applications in diagnosis of infections or disease processes. No longer the treatment of a disorder is guided by intuition and spot evaluation of symptoms. Rather the actual cause of any disorder can now be evaluated in greater detail, all thanks to development in many useful applications of immunology which in many diseases is the only known form of available diagnosis, e.g. transplantation medicine is based entirely on immunology.
- Some of the techniques which have found widespread usage are listed below.

A. TECHNIQUES INVOLVING ANALYSIS OF ANTIGEN-ANTIBODY INTERACTIONS

I. Immunodiffusion

Simple antigen-antibody reactions *in vitro* are detected by immunodiffusion techniques (ID). These techniques are extremely specific and can detect and quantify specific molecular structures even in the presence of contaminating molecules. The ID techniques are precipitation reactions in gels. When molecules such as soluble antigens diffuse from a homogenous solution into an agar gel containing a given concentration of antibody, the concentration of the antigen falls from a maximum at the solution - gel interface to zero at the leading edge of the region penetrated. Along this concentration gradient, at a point where the antigen concentration gives equivalence with a given concentration of antibody; a precipitate is formed. This region is called as zone of equivalence. This fact has been used since 1905 and developed into a range of highly sophisticated techniques. The following types of precipitation tests are in common use.

Single (simple) Immunodiffusion

1. *Oudin tube technique (one-dimensional):* This is a qualitative technique in which the antigen-antibody complexes form a precipitate in the region where antigen and antibody concentration is equivalent in gel matrix. They are used to detect the presence of an antigen(s) in sera, culture filtrates, tissue extracts or fractions from gradient centrifugation.
2. *Mancini's radial ID technique:*

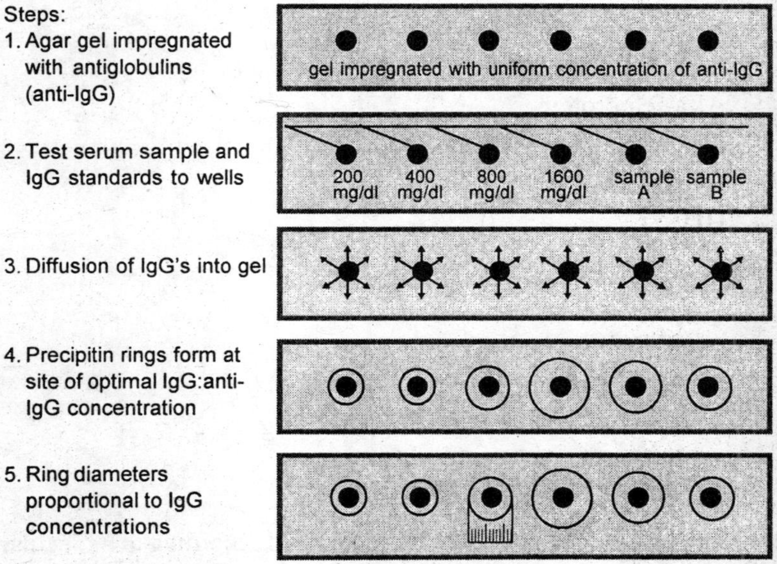

Figure 10.1: Radial immunodiffusion

Applications. Routinely used for estimating the concentration of various immunoglobulins such as IgG and IgM in agammaglobulinemia and multiple myeloma respectively. Also used to determine the concentration of transferrin and alfa fetoprotein (associated with certain liver tumors). One drawback to single radial immunodiffusion is the requirement of overnight incubation before reading the results. Sometimes you need the data more quickly (e.g., in determining failure of passive transfer for an individual animal).

II. ELISA (ENZYME-LINKED IMMUNOSORBENT ASSAY):

- The basic principle of an ELISA is to use an enzyme to detect the binding of Ag and Ab. The enzyme converts a colorless substrate (chromogen) to a colored product, indicating the presence of Ag:Ab binding. The detection depends on spectrophotometric assays.
- Presence of both antigen and antibodies in the clinical samples can checked using it.

Antigens

1. Alfa-fetoprotein
2. Human chorionic gonadotropin (hCG)
3. Hepatitis B
4. HIV

Antibodies

1. Anti-DNA antibodies
2. Anti-rubella antibodies
3. Anti-*Toxoplasma gondi* antibodies (Fig. 10.2)

III. WESTERN BLOTTING

In a western blot, antigens are first separated according to molecular weight by gel electrophoresis, then blotted onto a filter and developed using specific antibodies. The unique feature of the Western blot is

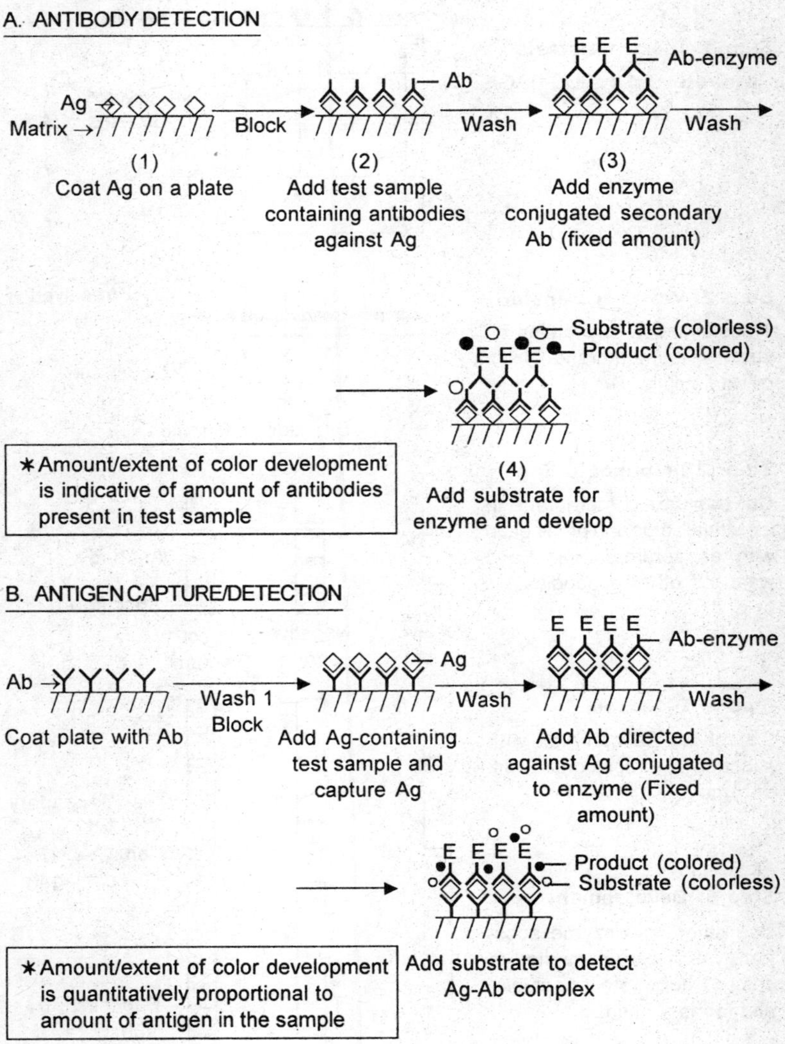

Figure 10.2: Representation of an ELISA to detect antibodies specific to Ag

that it identifies one or more individual Ags to which the Abs are bound. A positive sample will show binding of the enzyme-labeled antiglobulin at the particular sites where Ags of the infectious agent

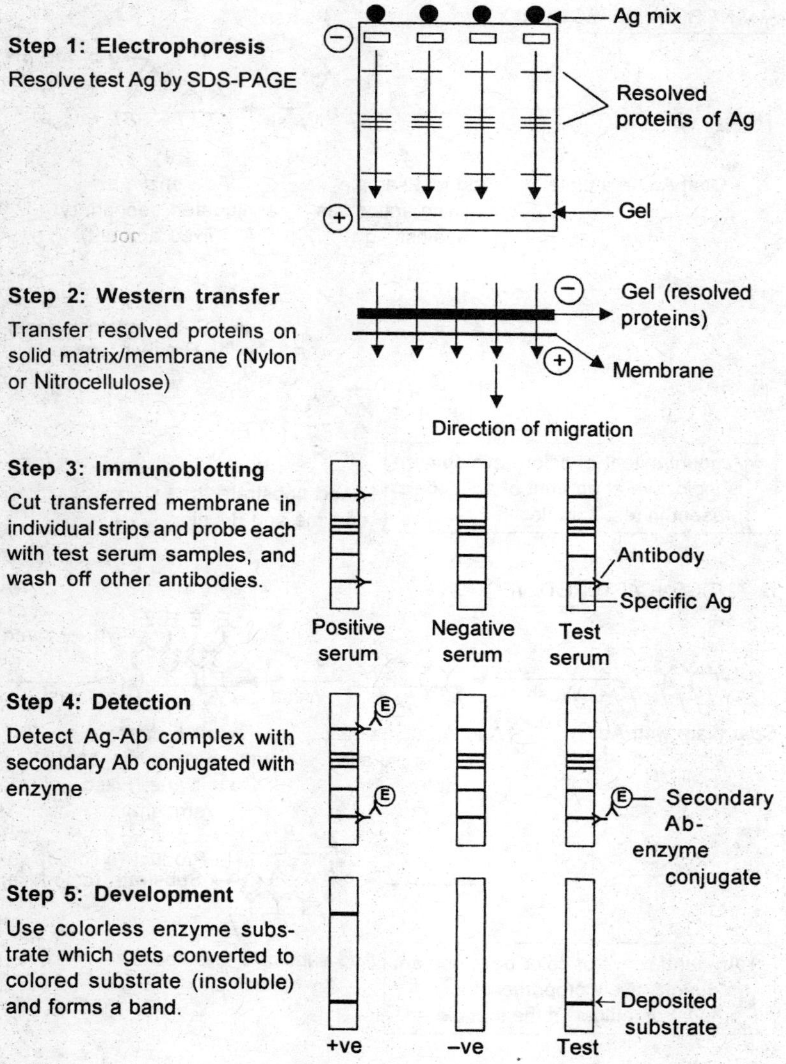

Figure 10.3: Western transfer and immunoblotting

are known to migrate in electrophoresis. If there is binding at other sites, the sample is considered negative because the binding is to a contaminating Ag in the preparation (Fig 10.3).

IV. RADIOIMMUNOASSAY (RIA)

RIA is an important technique in clinical biochemistry for estimation of hormones, steroids and drugs which are present in very minute quantities and cannot be detected by the colorimetric or other reagent methods. The technique is based on the specificity of the antigen - antibody reaction.

- The basic principle of a radioimmunoassay (RIA) is the use of radiolabeled Abs or Ags to detect Ag:Ab reactions. The Abs or Ags are labeled with the ^{125}I (iodine-125) isotope, and the presence of Ag:Ab reactions is detected using a gamma counter.
- The presence of the hormone in the serum sample inhibits binding of the radiolabeled hormone. Thus, the amount of radioactivity present in the test is inversely proportional to the amount of hormone in the serum sample (Fig. 10.4). A standard curve using increasing amounts of known concentrations of the

Step 1 Coating

Coat filter/plate with fixed concentration of antibody (pure) directed against test antigen (e.g. Hormone)

Step 2 Interaction

Add test sample, positive and negative control samples to individual filter/wells coated with antibody and allow to interact

Step 3 Label addition

Add known amount of radiolabeled Ag to each setup and allow to interact

Step 4 Recording radioactivity and preparing result. Amount of radioactivity retained is inversely proportional to the concentration of hormone in sample

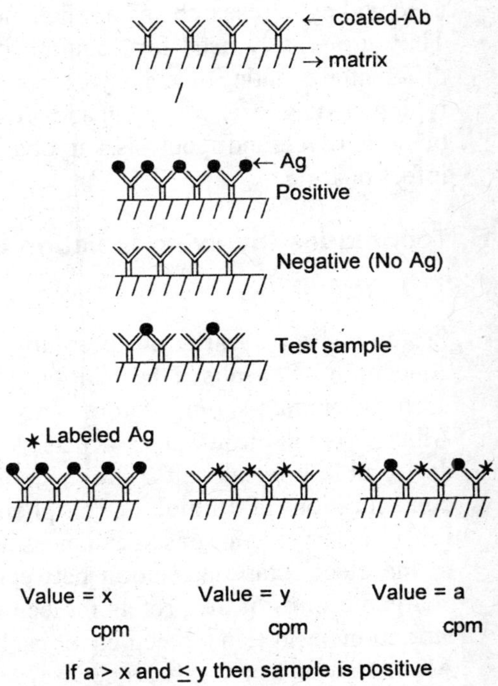

Figure 10.4: Principle of RIA

hormone is used to determine the quantity in the sample (Fig. 10.4).

- RIA finds applications in the measurement of peptide/steroid hormones such as T3, T4, TSH, hCG progesterone, etc. in clinical chemistry. RIAs are highly sensitive and quantitative, capable of detecting small amounts of Ag or Ab. As a result, they are often used to measure the quantities of hormones or drugs present in a patient's serum.
- Another use of the RIA is to measure the quantities of serum IgE antibodies specific for various allergens in a patient's serum.

V. FLUORESCENCE ACTIVATED CELL SORTER (FACS) AND IMMUNOFLUORESCENCE

- As multiple parameters-size, granularity, DNA or RNA content, DNA nucleotide ratios, cellular antigens and receptors, etc. can be measured using these instruments, they have come to be used widely in research and applied medicine.
- They are widely used for counting of blood cells including differential counting of leukocytes, isolating T- cell subsets, tissue typing, in diagnosis, treatment and prognosis in cancer, in study of the cell cycle and apoptosis, karyotyping, diagnosis of bacterial infections, etc.

B. Techniques Involving Isolation of Pure Antibodies

I. Salt Fractionation

- Proteins show a variation in solubility that depends on the concentration of salts in the solution. This method is frequently used to separate serum proteins into albumins and globulins. Albumin is soluble in water whereas globulins are not. Globulins are soluble in weak salt solutions, going into solution at salt concentrations of 0.1 mol/ L. This phenomenon called "Salting In" because presence of salt enhances the solubility. This is due to the electrostatic attraction between the salt ions and the charged groups of the protein molecules, which decreases the attraction of protein molecules for each other.
- Alternatively, as the salt concentration increases, the salt ions compete for the water molecules of the hydrated polar groups

of the proteins so that the proteins become dehydrated and less soluble-the phenomenon of "Salting Out", wherein the protein is brought out of solution by adding salt. Each protein has a characteristic salting out point based on the its characteristic water molecule requirement to maintain soluble status.

- Ammonium sulfate is most commonly used for salt fractionation and gamma globulins are generally precipitate out in 30-50 % ammonium sulfate.

II. Affinity Chromatography

- Affinity chromatography exploits the unique property of extremely specific biological interactions to achieve separation and purification. It makes use of specific affinity between the substance to be isolated and a molecule that it can specifically bind (a ligand). Thus, in theory affinity chromatography is capable of giving absolute purification, even from a complex mixture, in a single step.
- In principle these methods can be used to purify almost any macromolecule including enzymes, antibodies, specific and general classes of nucleic acids, vitamin binding proteins, repressors and other control elements.
- The technique requires that the material to be isolated is capable of reversibly binding to a specific ligand, attached to an insoluble matrix.

$$\underset{\text{Matrix}}{M} + \underset{\substack{\text{Ligand}\\\text{Attached to matrix}}}{L} \rightleftharpoons \underset{\text{complex}}{ML}$$

- Protein A, which is produced from staphylococcal cell walls has very high affinity for Fc portion of IgG molecules and hence can be used for purification of IgG fraction.

C. Techniques Involving Isolation of Lymphocyte populations

I. Ficoll-Isopaque Gradient

- Ficoll has a density greater than the lymphocytes but less than that of RBCs and granulocytes.

- When defibrinated blood is layered on Ficoll-Hypaque and centrifuged, the RBCs and PMNs pass though the ficoll to form a pellet at the bottom of the tube.
- The lymphocytes settle at the interface of the medium and Ficoll and they can be removed/ retrived from there.

II. FACS

- Based on the surface markers of various lymphocytes, various different types of lymphocytes can be separated using the marker specific antibody conjugated to a fluorophore.
- The number of cells isolated is, however, limited by the flow-rate of the sorter as individual cell is analyzed in this technique.

D. Techniques Involving Analysis of Effector Cells (Effector Cell Assays)

I. Plaque Forming Assays

- Antibody forming cells are analyzed by this assay wherein a test cell population (which is to be screened for antibody producing cells) is mixed with sensitized RBCs.
- Following incubation, the antibody-producing B-cells secrete antibody which after deposition on sensitized RBC leads to their lysis through a complement-mediated pathway forming clear zones or '*plaques*' in the culture dish.

II. ELISPOT Assay

- The technique is used to detect B-cell producing specific antibody or T-cells producing specific cytokines.
- The lymphocytes are plated on antigen or cytokine-sensitized plates. The secreted antibody or cytokine produced by either B-cell or T-cell respectively is then captured on the plate if secreted by the lymphocyte pool under analysis.
- The captured antibody or cytokine is then detected using another ab or cytokine–antibody coupled with an colorimetric enzyme. Development of color indicates towards the presence of specific secretory cell in the lymphocyte population.

III. Lymphocyte Transformation/ Proliferation/ Stimulation Test

- The test relies on the ability of antigen to elicit proliferation of lymphocytes upon activation.
- If the antigen is not recognized then no proliferation of the cells is observed.
- In the test, the lymphocytes separated from the whole blood are mixed with test antigen and ^3H labeled thymidine and incubated for 16 hours in culture media.
- If antigen causes stimulation, then lymphocyte population will proliferate and divide consequently taking up the ^3H thymidine (analog for DNA synthesis).
- The cells are then harvested on a glass filter and the retained radioactivity is measured in liquid scintillation counting. Uptake of H thymidine indicated by radioactivity retention by cells indicates towards the sensitivity of the lymphocytes to the antigen.

Index

H

I

L

M

O

P

R

S

T